"One of the great cover freedom a the release of Stc ing are evident th combination of biblical insights from Scripture and real-life stories of redemption. *Stay Here* will equip many to access the healing power and fullness of life that are promised to every person through Jesus."

Bill Johnson, senior leader of Bethel Church, Redding, CA,
and author of *Born for Significance* and *God is Good*

"I am grateful for Jacob's friendship, commitment to the gospel, and the mission of Stay Here. This part of the book really needs to be shouted from the rooftops: 'It's okay to not to be okay, but it's not okay to stay that way.' I'm glad that I chose to not stay that way; I'm glad that I chose to stay here."

Joshua Broome, co-founder of Share the King;
husband, father, preacher, and author

"Suicide is a modern-day plague that has stained an entire generation. I have met countless students who have attempted suicide, and countless more who know friends whose stories ended too soon. In *Stay Here*, my friend Jacob Coyne writes a call to action that all of us can be part of. Whether this is part of your story or not, I can assure you it has touched every teenager and twentysomething you know. Read this book as a lifeline. Read it to understand. Read this to join a movement of those standing in the gap for this generation to STAY HERE!"

Nick Hall, evangelist and founder of Pulse
and the Together movement

"For too long, many have remained silent about the battle taking place in countless lives. That is why *Stay Here* is such a needed message. My friend Jacob Coyne shares with authenticity and authority about the impact of mental health, suicide, and the hope that is available to every person through Jesus."

Tyler Sollie, Life Center Church

"*Stay Here* by Jacob Coyne is a powerful book that exposes the lies of suicide and offers help to anyone who has struggled with their mental health. With honesty and compassion, Jacob shares his own journey of overcoming depression and finding hope in Christ. This book is a must-read for anyone seeking to overcome the darkness of suicidal thoughts and discover the light of hope and healing."

Pastor Mike Signorelli, lead pastor of V1 Church

"There is no one I know with a more anointed and authoritative message around setting Gen Z free from suicide and depression than Jacob Coyne. This book is timely, powerful, and needed."

Grant Skeldon, Next Gen director at THINQ;
author of *The Passion Generation*

"Jacob Coyne and Stay Here are leading the way in lifting a spirit of death off an entire generation. In a world where suicide rates are ever on the rise, *Stay Here* offers a message of hope and healing for all those fighting against the darkness of anxiety, depression, and despair. At the turn of every page, we hear echoes of the Savior Himself: 'I have come that they may have LIFE, and life to the full.'"

Colby Maier, pastor of Bloom church

"There are few people I admire as much as my brother Jacob. His heart to see generations free from suicide and mental health issues is provoking. I know his book *Stay Here* will bring freedom to the heart of every reader. A mental health revival is on the horizon."

Jonah Coyne, co-founder of Stay Here and central student pastor of Gateway Church

"In *Stay Here*, Jacob gives us a needed message for this generation. He has a unique way of confronting the reality of the challenges we face while standing firm in the hope of Jesus. I can't encourage you enough to read this book and buy it for others. It is transformational."

Jessika Tate, founder and president of Yielded Ministries

"Jacob's message is the way through anxiety and depression. It's okay not to be okay, but you don't have to stay that way. I find so much hope in the pages of this book, and you can too."

Rebekah Lyons, bestselling author of *Rhythms of Renewal*

"Jacob Coyne is one of our generation's greatest encouragers on the topic of soul care and mental health. 'Stay here' is his life message, and throughout this book, you'll discover that Jesus sees your internal struggle more clearly than anyone, yet he loves you more than anyone."

Judah Smith, lead pastor of Churchome

"It's concerning to witness the mental health crisis that has engulfed a generation. Social media and constant comparison have left them grappling with negative effects. They've been crying for help, but we've been ignoring their pleas for too long. Thankfully, Jacob has stepped up with a powerful message—Stay here!—reminding them of their significance. It's time for us to act, and I am deeply grateful that this book inspires us to do so."

Becky Johnson, executive pastor of Jesus Culture Sacramento

Stay Here

Stay Here

Uncovering God's Plan to Restore Your Mental Health

Jacob Coyne

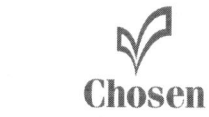

Chosen
a division of Baker Publishing Group
Minneapolis, Minnesota

© 2023 by Jacob Coyne

Published by Chosen Books
Minneapolis, Minnesota
www.chosenbooks.com

Chosen Books is a division of
Baker Publishing Group, Grand Rapids, Michigan

Printed in the United States of America

All rights reserved. No part of this publication may be reproduced, stored in a retrieval system, or transmitted in any form or by any means—for example, electronic, photocopy, recording—without the prior written permission of the publisher. The only exception is brief quotations in printed reviews.

ISBN 978-0-8007-6356-5 (trade paper)
ISBN 978-1-4934-4254-6 (ebook)
ISBN 978-0-8007-3000-0 (casebound)

Library of Congress Control Number: 2023010163

Unless otherwise identified, Scripture quotations are from The Holy Bible, English Standard Version® (ESV®), copyright © 2001 by Crossway, a publishing ministry of Good News Publishers. Used by permission. All rights reserved. ESV Text Edition: 2016

Scripture quotations identified CSB have been taken from the Christian Standard Bible®, copyright © 2017 by Holman Bible Publishers. Used by permission. Christian Standard Bible® and CSB® are federally registered trademarks of Holman Bible Publishers.

Scripture quotations identified GNT are from the Good News Translation in Today's English Version-Second Edition. Copyright © 1992 by American Bible Society. Used by permission.

Scripture quotations identified NIV are from THE HOLY BIBLE, NEW INTERNATIONAL VERSION®, NIV® Copyright © 1973, 1978, 1984, 2011 by Biblica, Inc.® Used by permission. All rights reserved worldwide.

Scripture quotations identified NKJV are from the New King James Version®. Copyright © 1982 by Thomas Nelson. Used by permission. All rights reserved.

Scripture quotations identified NLT are taken from the Holy Bible, New Living Translation, copyright © 1996, 2004, 2015 by Tyndale House Foundation. Used by permission of Tyndale House Publishers, Inc., Carol Stream, Illinois 60188. All rights reserved.

Scripture quotations identified KJV are from the King James Version of the Bible.

Baker Publishing Group publications use paper produced from sustainable forestry practices and post-consumer waste whenever possible.

23 24 25 26 27 28 29   7 6 5 4 3 2 1

To my wife, Mariah:
Thank you for staying with me
through my darkest nights.
Your love and prayers
helped pull me through.
I love you so much.

To my family:
Together, we're turning
our pain into purpose,
and it's changing thousands of lives.
I couldn't do this without you.

To anyone struggling with
finding reasons to keep going:
I pray this book will be your sign to live.

In memory of Greg Sweet,
my uncle and incredible friend.

Contents

Foreword by Nick Vujicic 11

1. This Is Your Sign to Live 15
2. The Way Is Through 27
3. It's Okay to Not Be Okay, but It's Not Okay to Stay That Way 41
4. How Free Do You Want to Be? 61
5. When Anxiety Attacks 79
6. Tired of Being Tired 95
7. The Prison Cell of Anger 109
8. Stuck in the Loop of Stinking Thinking 119
9. Jesus Can Heal Your Trauma 133
10. Gen Z Will Be Suicide Free 143

Personal Prayer Starters 159
Stay Here Resources 165
Acknowledgments 167
Notes 169

Foreword

Growing up, I could not imagine living my whole life without arms and legs. I didn't understand why God would allow me to be born this way. I worried that I would never be able to have a job or be independent. I assumed having a wife and my own family was not in the cards for me. So many fears plagued my mind. The bullying I faced and the fear of being alone kept me in a dark depression and brought me to a suicide attempt when I was just ten years old. At that time, I did not think I could live without arms and legs.

If you told me back then the ways that God was going to use my life, I would not have believed you. Today, I have a beautiful wife and four amazing children. I've traveled the world, and God has given me platforms to inspire and encourage millions of brokenhearted people. I have had the privilege of meeting with presidents and leaders of nations. Despite the challenges I have faced, God has been faithful to turn my pain into purpose.

Foreword

If you have battled with mental health, I want you to know that you're not alone. Maybe you've thought about suicide or even attempted it. But the fact that you decided to open this book tells me that you haven't given up. You have chosen to keep fighting for today because deep down, you know you were created for a greater purpose. Maybe you haven't seen what that purpose is yet, but something in your heart tells you there is more. I want you to know that I am proud of you.

I gave my life to Christ at the age of fifteen. I asked God to give me arms and legs, but I also decided that even if He didn't, I needed Him to rescue me from the two biggest disabilities: sin and death. Even if I didn't get the miracle I was hoping for, I asked Him to help me be a miracle for someone else. I wanted my life to mean something. I could have stayed angry and bitter about my circumstances and taken matters into my own hands, but that would have led to a life much less than the purpose God intended. Or worse, I could have ended my life. But let my story be evidence to you that when we give God our brokenness, He always makes something beautiful.

God has dreams for you better than anything you have imagined. Jeremiah 29:11 says, "'For I know the plans I have for you,' declares the LORD, 'plans to prosper you and not to harm you, plans to give you hope and a future'" (NIV). If you are overwhelmed about your life, remember these words. I used to worry about my future without arms and legs. Looking back, I can see that God always had my best interests in mind. We don't have to know the whole

Foreword

plan. Trust that God has given you everything you need for today to take the next step.

I recently had the chance to interview Jacob Coyne for our Champions for the Brokenhearted series. It is evident that Jacob carries the burden of our heavenly Father to see Gen Z (and the generations that come after) live. I believe that he is a trailblazer for this generation to find their true identity in Christ. I pray that as you read this book, you will see the truth about who God says you are, and see His heart for you. I do not know what you have been through, but I know the God who does. You may not be able to see anything from where you are right now, but keep going. There are others, like Jacob, who have been through the dark valley and are standing strong on the other side, cheering you on. Keep fighting the good fight of faith. What is crushing you right now can become a powerful testimony that changes the world! I implore you today to choose life. Take one day at a time. You are an overcomer. You have a great story to tell. I love you, and I believe in you. Stay here!

— Nick Vujicic, founder of Life Without Limbs ministry

1

This Is Your Sign to Live

Our world is in the middle of a mental health crisis. Anxiety, depression, and suicide rates are at all-time highs. Let me put it to you this way: As of this writing, every forty seconds, someone takes their own life. That means that by the time you're done reading this chapter, more than twenty people will have died by suicide.[1] And if you were to read this book from cover to cover in one sitting, 9,756 people would have taken their own lives around the globe during that time.[2]

These aren't just nameless, faceless statistics. These are people—your friends and neighbors at school, work, and church. Twelve-year-olds, seventeen-year-olds, and thirty-four-year-olds. High school class presidents. Athletes and artists. Daughters and sons. And they matter.

Does it break your heart to watch this happen to your generation—to any generation? Does it hurt when you see this? It should, because this is not the way things are meant to be. If we have breath in our lungs, if our heart is beating, we matter to God. He is a God of life, and He has destined every soul on this planet to physically live this life to the fullest. Do you believe that?

How do I know this is true? Because the Bible says God desires that none should perish (2 Peter 3:9). None means zero. We're all intended to know the heart of God, our heavenly Father, and His heart wants us all to know the love of Jesus Christ.

In this book I'll ask you some challenging questions to propel you not only to seek and find healing for your own soul but to then bring healing to the brokenhearted all around you. Your generation depends on you to live and bring life to the hardest and darkest places. Because if not you, then who? And if not now, then when? If you're a teenager, who else will bring Jesus to your school or college? Who else will pray for your friends? Will you do it? We must. We are the last line of defense for the broken.

The Bible tells us the enemy has come to steal, kill, and destroy, and I know the world seems dark and hopeless all around us. But I have good news from that same passage in Scripture. Jesus Christ is shouting loud and clear, "I have come to bring life and life to the fullest!" (John 10:10, paraphrased).

I long to see self-hatred, self-harm, and certainly anxiety, depression, and suicide lifted off our world, especially among the younger generations. Though suicide may currently be the second leading cause of death around the globe, here's more good news: <u>it's the most preventable cause of death</u>. So what's keeping us from preventing it? What's keeping us from ending this epidemic? It's been inaction, it's been our silence, and it's been our lack of prayer.

This Ends Now

I ask you to join me in saying "<u>This ends now</u>." We will pray. We will take action. We will reach out. We will share the good news of Jesus that saves broken and hurting souls. Jesus is with us in this battle, and we will win.

Here is a story to encourage you, to let those of you who need a sign to live know that there is always hope, and to let those of you ready to fight the battle for others know it's easier to save someone from suicide than you think.

In 2020, I started a nonprofit mental health organization called Stay Here, and we came up with a wild and bold vision: *Gen Z will be suicide free.* (Gen Z's age range is anyone born from 1996 to 2012.) Our organization spreads awareness through our clothing line, and we offer a crisis chat line, counseling, and free suicide prevention training and certification online.

In 2021, we came out with T-shirts emblazoned with our vision statement—*Gen Z will be suicide free*—in bold red ink. A friend named Jocelyn wore one of these shirts to a Seattle Mariners baseball game, and little did she know that a nineteen-year-old young woman there was planning to kill herself that very night, after the game. But she'd bought a ticket to this event literally hoping to find *a sign to live*.

Somehow, by the providence of God and in the midst of thousands of people, the two crossed paths, and the message on Jocelyn's T-shirt stopped this hurting soul in her tracks. She walked up to Jocelyn and asked, "What is this shirt all about? What does it mean?" Jocelyn told her about the gospel of Jesus Christ, and after one conversation, this teenager said, "I was going to kill myself tonight, but this is my sign to live."

Maybe you're hurting and battling suicidal thoughts just like that young woman was. You might be thinking you're all alone in your storm and beyond saving. But again, I'm telling you there's hope. Someone has been reading your journal entries. Someone has seen you in your lowest moments alone in your bedroom. His name is Jesus, and He's here to set you free.

Let this book be your sign to live. My prayer is that you will find the healing and freedom you've been desperately crying out for, you'll experience wholeness, and you'll even become a sign to live for others around you. If you're a follower of Jesus, you carry the resurrection life of Jesus in your veins. You will not die; you will live. And you will tell the world about what God has done in your life.

I will fight for the born who wish they had not been born.

I will fight for the living who wish they were dead.

I will fight for the breathing who wish they were without breath.

Let me fight for you as you read these pages, and then, when you're ready, please join me in the fight for your generation.

How I Got Here

Let me tell you how I got into this fight in the first place. Few people wake up one morning and say, "I think my calling in life is to stop suicide." But suicide is a heavy topic, and I was led to this place because heavy things happened to me and around me. Oftentimes our deepest pain can lead us into our purpose, and soon it became an injustice for me to keep sitting around without taking action.

A few years ago, my uncle Greg Sweet took his own life. Greg wasn't just a relative I saw only during the holidays. He was a father figure and a mentor to me. He was also a father to his four incredible girls. Greg always took the spotlight in any room he walked into. He was loud, joyful, an includer, and a lover of anything that required risk. He possessed a deep love for God and constantly sang worship songs in a '90s-grunge sort of style.

Unfortunately, Greg was diagnosed with Parkinson's disease, and it took a great toll on his go-getter lifestyle. After he'd battled the illness for about six years, it began to affect his mind as well as his body. And then, unexpectedly, he took his own life in the late summer of 2015.

Saying goodbye to Greg in the hospital was one of the hardest things I've ever had to do. On many days memories of him come to mind, causing my eyes to quickly fill with tears. My uncle never got to meet my three daughters. He isn't here to cheer me on like he used to. It hurts. Greg's death put a fire in my soul, a flame of anger toward mental illness and suicide.

Greg isn't the only one I lost to suicide. When I was a youth pastor, two of my students took their own lives. And then the last straw for me came in 2019, when my friend Jarrid Wilson died by suicide on World Suicide Prevention Day. Jarrid was a great husband, father, and pastor. When pastors take their own lives, you know something has gone terribly wrong with the mental well-being of our culture.

Before Jarrid took his life, I had a recurring dream that still marks me today. In the dream, Jarrid and I were walking along a beach in Southern California, talking like usual. But then a strange thing happened: a bubble of water formed all around Jarrid's head, and he was drowning on dry ground. I was concerned and asked if I could help him, but he kept telling me everything was fine as he ignored the fact that he was drowning.

I don't believe in coincidences, so I knew God was trying to tell me something about Jarrid through that dream. But I never had enough courage to ask my friend about it. I never called him to see if he was okay. I'd had disturbing dreams about my uncle Greg too, and I'd never checked on him either. Why didn't I? For the same reason. Because I was afraid.

I was afraid I'd offend them. I was afraid I'd hurt their feelings. And I believed the myth that said asking someone whether they're experiencing severe depression and might be contemplating suicide could make the situation worse or even plant the thought of suicide into their mind. I was afraid that asking them about my dream might actually push them off a mental ledge.

But after Jarrid died, I spent hours upon hours researching self-harm, mental illness, and suicide. I discovered that asking a simple question such as "Have you had thoughts of suicide lately?" can actually save a life and is more helpful than hurtful.

Three Lies of Suicide

Before I go on with my story, let's talk about three myths of suicide we know are often at play. They're all based on the enemy's lies, and if he's speaking them to you, fight back!

1. Lie: Everyone will be better off if you're gone.

The enemy tells depressed people that everyone will be better off when they're gone. Kurt Cobain wrote a long goodbye letter. At the end of it, he wrote to his wife, Courtney, these words: "Please keep going Courtney, for Frances [sic]." Frances is their daughter. "For her life, which will be so much happier without me."[3] I wonder if Frances's life is better without her father. I can't answer that; only she can. But it's most likely that taking your life won't be better for anyone.

So don't believe the lie that you're a burden, that when you make the choice to leave, everyone else will be better off. No one will be better off. Those you love will live out their lives with guilt, a cloud of trauma, self-doubt, questions, pain, and anger for the rest of their lives. And all the while they'll think they weren't worth fighting for. Oh, they'll know it wasn't you who took your life. They'll know it was the darkness ravaging you, that you really weren't thinking clearly. They'll know that intellectually. But it will be a gut punch in their soul, and it will be agonizing.

2. Lie: Suicide is your destiny.

Suicide is not God's purpose, and it's not His plan for you. Your destiny is not in leaving; it's in staying. Yes, you may be free from your earthly pain, but you'll be leaving your true destiny behind. You were handcrafted by God on purpose, for a purpose. It's not about what life has done to you; it's about what you can do to life. Remember this verse? "I know the plans I have for you, declares the LORD, plans for welfare and not for evil, to give you a future and a hope" (Jeremiah 29:11).

3. Lie: Suicide is glamorous.

This is shocking, I know. You say, *How could suicide be glamorous?* Well, the enemy has a way of making terrible things look that way. Scientists dub one way "suicide contagion." Comedian Robin Williams took his own life, and in the four months that followed, the suicide rate in America rose 10 percent, and the manner of his suicide rose more than 30 percent. Going back decades, actress Marilyn Monroe reportedly took her own life, and the suicide rate rose 12 percent.[4]

In some crazy way, the media attention for some celebrities who commit suicide adds to their legacy. It creates a cult effect, a vortex that sucks people in and pulls them under to this glamour, making them believe suicide is actually a good thing.

If you're having suicidal thoughts, don't let these powerful myths sway you. They're lies. As I said, fight back! Stay here. We're here for you. And we can help.

The Birth of Stay Here

The revelation that asking others about their mental health can help rather than harm brought me, along with my extended family, to the point of starting Stay Here in 2020. We wanted to break the stigma around mental illness and suicide and change statistics.

From the end of 2019 to the spring of 2020, I had spoken in a couple of high schools on the topic of suicide and mental illness with great results. We had bookings through to the end of 2020, and lives were being changed. But then COVID-19 hit and took away all our bookings. Sadly, when people needed help more than ever, we couldn't physically be there to bring it to them.

But we couldn't allow the pandemic to keep us from bringing hope to the hurting, so we prayed, brainstormed, and developed a new plan. Instead of Stay Here consisting of a couple of people with microphones speaking at schools, what if we trained and equipped millions of leaders to reach their own homes, schools, workplaces, teams, churches, and cities?

Well, in April 2021, that's exactly what began to happen after God gave me a life-changing vision. My wife, Mariah, and I were attending a leaders retreat in Kona, Hawaii, when at one point a dozen pastors circled us to pray for us and our ministry. During this powerful time of prayer, I had a vision. I saw a stadium full of teenagers with their hands raised. On the stage was a man of God named Lou Engle leading the entire stadium in prayer for their generation to be saved, and then he shouted the phrase "Gen Z will be suicide free!" The crowd shouted the phrase back and then marched out of the stadium and onto their campuses, shouting it in the hallways and classrooms.

I knew what God was showing me: If we really wanted to save lives, we needed an army. It couldn't be done with just a couple of motivational speakers. As I already shared, we put *Gen Z will be suicide free* on T-shirts, and now thousands of people wear them all over the world. Anytime I'm traveling, I see one in an airport or at the event where I'm speaking. The message is truly spreading.

A few months later, our team developed a free online (or in-person) suicide prevention training that anyone can take. We call it the ACT Training, where you can learn how to save a life after spotting the warning signs of someone battling depression, anxiety, and even suicidal thoughts. We published the training in August 2021, and a year later, as of this writing, more than fifteen thousand people have completed the course.

I tell you all this to let you know that people do care. Help is on the way, and this generation—Gen Z—will choose life. The future is bright for us. And I believe thousands of other mental health organizations will start up over the next decade and join us in the fight to save lives. Those who are suffering will learn help is available, including from professionals in the medical and counseling fields. As I indicate later in this book, all plans that lead to mental health healing are God's plans, for we're told that every good and perfect thing comes from Him (James 1:17).

But most of all, help is available from Jesus Himself. Always.

Will you join me in choosing life? Will you fight for those who don't want to see another day? Together, we can be the sign the Gen Z generation is searching for. We can shine a light into the dark places. We can breathe fresh purpose into weary souls. We can change the narrative over this generation.

Are you in?

Prayer

Jesus, I choose life. I'm ready to receive the life you promised me, a rich and full one. I'm also ready to be a carrier of life to the brokenhearted. Let your light shine not only in me but through me to the darkest places. Let me be a sign to live for those looking for one. Give me hope for my own life and for the future of the Gen Z generation. In your name, amen.

For Reflection

1. What do you think God's plan is for your generation? When you think about your generation, do you have hope? Or are you struggling to see a brighter future? Ask God to help you see what He sees.

2. As you read this book, will you be willing to ask God to bring change into your own life? Are you ready for transformation and healing? If so, in your own words, ask God to start that process now.

2

The Way Is Through

We're Going on a Bear Hunt is one of my favorite books to read to my kids, but its story is actually pretty strange and weird. A mom and dad and their kids and their dog decide to spend the day looking for a bear. (Like, who does that? Don't ever *look* for a bear.)

On their journey, they find all these obstacles. Like mud. A river. A snowstorm. A forest. A cave. Tall, wavy grass. But every time this family encounters one of these hindrances, they decide they just have to go through it, because they can't get past it any other way.

We're Going on a Bear Hunt can teach us a lesson or two when it comes to obstacles we all experience in our lives. We try to avoid (or ignore) anxiety, depression, sadness, or grief. But the more we try, the bigger they become, at least under the surface. Have you ever experienced that? The more you try to run in the opposite direction, or the more you quote Scripture, or the more you ask God to just deliver you out of your situation, the bigger the problem becomes.

King David even knew this. In Psalm 23:4 he said to God, "Even though I walk *through* the valley of the shadow of death, I will fear no evil, for you are with me" (emphasis added). He knew that when he was in the valley, he had to go through it. And just like King David and the family in *We're Going on a Bear Hunt*, you have to go through your valleys—through life's obstacles—too. It's necessary to get to the mountain.

The beauty of that journey, though, is this: Arriving at the mountain is so much sweeter because God was with you not just in the victory of the mountain but in the pain of the valley.

Let's Be Real

One of the biggest lies we hear in Christianity today is that God is with us only on the mountain. That He's with us only when the praise is right. Only when we're fasting and praying. Only when we're quoting the Scriptures. Only when we're all full of faith. But God is with us in the valley too.

Why do we believe that lie? Because we're in a social media generation. We think that just like we show only our highlights to others on social media and network sites like Instagram, TikTok, YouTube, Facebook, and LinkedIn, we need to show God only our highlights. We think He doesn't want to see our pain, our mess, our ugly days. Just like the rest of the world, right?

I'm sure you aren't posting photos of your dirty laundry or your dirty house on Instagram, are you? No. You guys are fluffing your pillows, making sure your living room's looking nice and pristine for the background of your new selfie. And then ten minutes later, everything looks like junk again.

But God doesn't want just your highlights. He doesn't want only your good days. He wants everything. He wants it all. So let's throw out the lie that God meets us only on the mountain. The Bible says the arm of the Lord is not too short to save (Isaiah 59:1). Why does His arm need to be long? So He can reach us in the lowest valley. We've got to stop believing that He meets us only on mountain peaks. God met with Moses on the mountain, but His heart was also grieved for the people of Israel when they made an idol of a golden cow and worshipped it. God reached down to them. He loved them too.

I don't know any hero of the faith in Scripture who didn't go through some kind of challenge. Do you? Let's start with Hannah, for example.

Hannah

Hannah constantly cried tears over her barrenness, desperate for God to give her a son. How long must she have been crying? How many miscarriages did she have? Only God knows. But she cried. And she wept. And she prayed that God would provide for her a son.

And God did. He gave her Samuel, a prophet of God who spoke in the midst of silence. During that time period, God wasn't speaking to anyone, because no one was listening. Everyone was so disobedient to Him. But in the midst of the spiritual barrenness of Israel and the physical barrenness of Hannah's womb, God gave this woman a prophet. Hannah had just wanted a son, but God gave her an incredible man of God in that son. And this man anointed Saul, the first king of Israel, and then King David. Jesus came from the line of King David. What a miracle happened to Hannah.

Elijah

What about Elijah? Elijah had a mountaintop experience. Can you imagine being the guy who was so bold to say that God would show up and bring fire from heaven in front of the prophets of Baal? Elijah mocked the false prophets of this foreign god as fire from heaven came down on the altar. He was a hero of Israel. He proved to everyone that there's only one God.

But moments later, he heard Queen Jezebel consider him a dead man. And then guess what Elijah did after that mountaintop experience? He ran. He'd just witnessed one of the most profound miracles we see in Scripture, God showed up for him, but he still ran in terror from the evil queen. He retreated to the desert and even asked God to kill him. He was suicidal.

The beauty of this story is that God showed up for Elijah again, this time in the desert, when he was all alone, wanting to throw in the towel and die. God comforted him. God encouraged him. God refreshed him. God was with Elijah on the mountain and in the darkest valley.

Peter

And what about Peter? Oh, man, Peter. He said things to Jesus like, "Lord, I'll die with you. I'll go anywhere with you. I'm with you to the very end." And Jesus said, "You'll deny me three times." Peter does deny Jesus three times and then doesn't even have the boldness or the heart to show up and watch his friend be crucified. Can you imagine the shame, the grief Peter felt over not even being brave enough to come to the crucifixion after he'd denied Jesus?

And it gets worse. Three short days later, in his grief and anguish, Peter decided to quit being a disciple and go back to his old trade—being a fisherman. Where did Jesus find Peter after He rose from the dead? He found him fishing. He'd quit. He'd left his role as the "rock." He'd given up. But Jesus came to Peter in the man's shame, in his grief, in his brokenness. Jesus restored him.

Maybe you're like Peter. Maybe you've run back to your old ways. Maybe you've been faking it hoping you'll make it. You put on the holy roller smile at church, but in reality you're too tired to even reach out to God and His church for help.

But I'm telling you today: God is reaching out to you. His grace is reaching out to you. And we have to accept the fact that we can't make it on our own. This is what Paul tells us Jesus said to him: "My grace is sufficient for you, for my power is made perfect in weakness" (2 Corinthians

12:9). And then in that same verse, Paul writes, "Therefore I will boast all the more gladly of my weaknesses, so that the power of Christ may rest upon me."

It's time that we start boasting of our weaknesses. If you want God's power to be on your life, boast about your weaknesses, and boast about Christ's strength.

Jesus doesn't touch the strong; He reaches for the weak. He even said, "I didn't come for the healthy. I came for the sick." It's the sick who need a doctor. If you're feeling sick inside right now, or if you're physically sick, Jesus comes for you. He comes to those who can't come to Him. How about the crippled man at the pool of Bethesda in the book of John, chapter 5? He couldn't even stand. He couldn't do anything. But Jesus saw his brokenness and reached out to him. (We'll talk about this story more in chapter 4.)

Sometimes we don't even have the strength to reach out to God, but God is strong enough to reach out to us. That's what the cross is. It's God's outstretched arms to humanity because we can't reach Him. We can't do this on our own.

Your weakness is a magnet for God's strength, so stop hiding it. Stop hiding your weaknesses.

Let me tell you about my story of hiding weakness and how God brought me through a valley I was in.

The Worst Year of My Life

Let me introduce you to 2018, the absolute worst year of my life. All hell broke loose within thirty days in the month of June, and the effect on my mental health was intense.

The Way Is Through

It all started when Mariah found out she was pregnant with our second baby. We were so excited to build our family. We already had our daughter, River, and now another child was on the way! We told so many people and started taking pregnancy announcement photos. And we shopped at Babies R Us just before it went out of business, when everything was around 80 percent off. So we were, like, "Let's stock up for this new kiddo." We found an awesome crib and decided to buy it. I held Mariah's hand and looked into her eyes, laughing and smiling. And I remember the smile on her face and the glow in her eyes. She was so excited, and so was I.

But then we lost this baby at eleven weeks. Mariah had a miscarriage, and it broke our hearts in two.

That was the first loss.

Two weeks after that, we were in our backyard with friends and a bonfire when my stepdad called. He sounded so urgent. Something was wrong with my stepbrother.

"Jacob, I need you. Please get over to the house right now. Tucker's not okay. Tucker's not okay."

It was about a fifteen-minute drive, and when I got there, I saw police cars and an ambulance. I ran upstairs to Tucker's bedroom and watched as paramedics tried to resuscitate him. He'd relapsed, taking drugs he'd been free from for a good amount of time, his body not used to them now. He died right there in front of us, my stepdad holding him in his arms.

That was the second loss.

A few days later, Mariah and I were called into a mysterious emergency meeting for all staff at our church with only a one-day notice. Once there, we learned our lead pastor was being fired for moral failure and other sins—and it tore our staff and church apart.

That was the third loss. Again, all this happened within thirty days, during the month of June.

By this time, I was so weak. I often lost track of what day it was. I lost track of how many days in a row I just lay on our couch after Mariah and I had tucked River into bed. I wept and screamed into a pillow. I had no strength to reach out to God. I had nothing. I cried so hard I thought I was going to die. It was the most intense pain, the most intense grief. I couldn't function. I couldn't go to work. I couldn't go to meetings. I couldn't leave the house. I couldn't think. I didn't want to get out of bed half the time.

As much as I could, I tried to hide my weakness. God knew all about it, of course. So did my family. But I didn't know how I was going to get out of this pit. I didn't know how I was going to get free. I didn't know how I was going to move on.

Turning Point

One of those nights, I decided to give God a sacrifice of praise. I didn't want to do it, because it was painful, but I made my way into our prayer room and turned on some worship music. I got out my journal and then silently prayed, *God, I need you to speak to me so badly. Please speak to me. What are you saying? What are you doing? What are you going to do about all this?*

God's words to me were so sweet, and I saw a vision of Jesus crying with me. Some of us see Jesus as just this fiery-eyed, fiery-haired, glorious King, but He weeps with us when we weep. He's also the Man who wept in the garden of Gethsemane on His knees, on His face, crying out for humanity.

I saw Jesus fighting for me. I saw Him praying for me. And I heard Him whisper into my ear, "Jacob, I haven't left you." And then He said, "Jacob, my love is stronger than death." Those promises are also in the Bible, and I've personally read them so many times over the years. But when I heard them that night, something began to happen in me.

The crying got more intense, but then it was like I was riding on a roller coaster. The crying turned into absolute laughter. The pain turned to joy. Healing was on the horizon for me. I could see it for the first time in a while. Jesus was restoring hope within me.

I would love to tell you I was healed right then and everything was better after that. But like the family on a bear hunt, I had to keep going through. No other option would get me to the other side. But as I moved through this valley of pain, my perspective was different. I knew I wasn't alone. There is a God who weeps with us. He sees our weakness. He sees us. And He's reaching out with His long arm.

The Way Forward

Grief doesn't end in a day, so the next step was counseling. It was time to share the struggle. I told my wife, "I'll keep receiving God's love, but, Mariah, we're going to a counselor. And we need to find a Christian counselor."

And, man, the first time we met with the Christian counselor we found, I sat on her office couch and immediately started crying.

She said, "Wow. We've got someone who's ready!"

I said, "No, I'm crying because I'm not ready. This is super embarrassing. I'm a pastor. I'm a leader. I'm a Christian. Christians don't go to counseling."

And she's, like, "Oh, honey. Oh, man. How wrong you are. You're about to get ready."

A word about shame: The shame I felt going to that office is the spirit of mere religion that keeps you quiet, hiding in the shadows, hiding your weakness. The shame you feel confessing your sins to someone else is the spirit of religion. The shame you feel talking about how painful your day has been, how painful a valley is for you, is the spirit of religion. We need to be able to be open and real and honest in the church. So let's go there. Let's talk about the taboo things. Let's talk about mental health in the church.

We had sessions with our counselor for months, and then it got to the point where she was, like, "What do you guys want to talk about today? There's nothing much left to deal with." We were so whole after going and going and going that I think our last time we just talked about our kids. We were shooting the breeze. And that was our final appointment with our counselor. We left healed.

Again, I would love to tell you it's been all butterflies and fairy tales and waterfalls ever since. But I still have hard days. Who doesn't? Yet Jesus promised He would heal the sick, and going to that counselor gave me the tools I need to go through grief when it comes.

We also need to be bolder about reaching out to others when we notice their pain. Let me say again that two people close to me—my uncle Greg and my friend Jarrid—committed suicide after I'd had disturbing dreams about them. And whispered warnings had been in my ear for months when I was awake: *Something's wrong. You should reach out, Jacob. You should ask him if he's depressed or even suicidal. You should take him out to coffee. Do something.*

For both of those men, though, I failed to reach out because I thought it was too awkward or even dangerous to bring up those concerns. But again, the truth about depression or suicide or grief is that bringing up the topic actually brings an avenue—an open door—to healing, not a danger of pushing them into suicide.

Man of Sorrows

I'm just going to break it to you. Jesus never once promised that we wouldn't have to go through grief. Even Jesus went through grief. Jesus wept. He went through grief when He saw unbelief. He no doubt went through grief when He lost His earthly father, Joseph. He went through grief when He looked at Israel and saw their rebellion against God. He went through grief in the garden of Gethsemane. The Bible says He was so overtaken by this grief and sorrow that His sweat was like drops of blood on the ground.

Maybe it's time for you to meet the man of sorrows. We love to talk about Jesus, the man who was anointed with the oil of joy beyond any of His companions. Yes, Jesus is the happiest person ever. But He also mourns with those who mourn. He experiences sorrow with those who are in the middle of sorrow. He sees our pain and knows our pain.

Maybe you think Jesus can't relate to your pain and your story. But look at the cross. Think about the wounds on His back when He was flogged. Think about the crown of thorns placed on His head, the slaps and the punches He took. But He knows what all pain feels like, because His pain wasn't just physical. The pain He felt on His way to the cross was your pain. He did this for you. Let this grief into the hands of the man of sorrows, and He will lead you through this valley. He will pour out the oil of joy on you as you get through this pain.

Whatever you're carrying—whether it's grief from a lost loved one; grief from a divorce or breakup; or grief from your own sin, depression, or anxiety—Jesus will sit with you. Right in the middle of this valley. He'll put His arm around you. He'll weep with you. He'll cry with you and then pull you through.

In Psalm 23:5-6, David says to God—as can we—"You prepare a table before me in the presence of my enemies; you anoint my head with oil; my cup overflows. Surely goodness and mercy shall follow me all the days of my life, and I shall dwell in the house of the LORD forever."

God wants to do that for you today. If you're hurting, if you have grief in your heart, if you're experiencing shame, I want to introduce you to the man of sorrows. He will heal you. He will restore you. He will redeem you. He sets every captive who comes to Him free. Isaiah 53:3 says, "He was despised and rejected by men, a man of sorrows and acquainted with grief." He knows your grief. Verses 3 and 4 go on to say, "And as one from whom men hide their faces he was despised, and we esteemed him not. Surely he has borne our griefs and carried our sorrows."

You've got to begin to let go of your grief and sorrow and place them into Jesus' arms. The Bible says He bore your grief on that cross. He carried your sorrow. He carried that depression. He carried that trauma. He carried that suicidal thought. He carried your addiction.

It's time that you stop carrying this thing on your own. Verses 4 and 5 in the same passage in Isaiah say, "We esteemed him stricken, smitten by God, and afflicted. But he was pierced for our transgressions; he was crushed for our iniquities; upon him was the chastisement that brought us peace, and with his wounds we are healed."

It's time to go through the valley with Jesus. I promise you, He will carry you through.

Prayer

I give my pain to you, Lord. You are the Healer. I give you my sadness, my sorrows. In my sorrows, you are the man of joy, and I trust that laughter and freedom come after this. I thank you for walking with me through this valley and that I'm not alone. You are with me in this place right now.

Jesus, whisper in my ear how much you love me, how you see me, how you know me, how you're going to bring me through. Reveal your face to me. Reveal your love. Reveal your heart. You bring life where there was death.

You bring light where there was darkness. You make all things new. Thank you, Father. Amen.

For Reflection

1. What memories you believe God wants to address with you came up as you read this chapter?
2. What parts of your present hurt or your past still hurt?
3. Are you ready to let Jesus walk you through this valley? Talk to Him about that right now.

3

It's Okay to Not Be Okay, but It's Not Okay to Stay That Way

We live in strange times. Some of you don't realize this because you weren't alive in any past generation, but the battles we all face today didn't even exist in the generation before us. I'm referring to the prevalence of available technology and what we can access and be exposed to. For instance, today almost any photo or video can be easily viewed on a smartphone, and much of what's available is offered for profit regardless of its lack of moral value.

Annually, the porn industry makes thirteen thousand films and close to $25 billion in profit, outpacing Hollywood's roughly six hundred movie releases with $10 billion in profit. It makes more money than Major League

Baseball, the NFL, and the NBA combined. And according to statistics, porn sites get more visitors each month than one of the world's top streaming sites (Netflix), one of its top shopping sites (Amazon), and one of its top social media sites (Twitter) combined.[1]

Social media app TikTok has one billion monthly active users worldwide, and 51 percent of them are Gen Z.[2] As of this writing, it's been the most downloaded app for the past two years. Gen Z also spends half of their waking hours on their phones with an average of 7.4 hours of screen time per day watching videos![3]

Scientists tell us—and I'm sure you agree—that we are collectively addicted to technology. And due to this addiction, our relational skills are dwindling. Families are splitting up. Kids are left to fend for themselves and grow up far faster than the generations before them. Statistically—especially because of social media—anxiety has entered nearly every home. Online, we all live in a fishbowl of constant comparison. And even if we wanted to, we can't escape a world where trolls and bullies are lurking in every corner of the internet.

So, then, it's no wonder that in study after study we read that teens and young people in their twenties are battling depression at unprecedented rates. Mental illness is a reality, and it's complex. But it's here, and it's in all our faces. If you're in the middle of this storm, you already know that's true.

Mental illness is not a one-size-fits-all problem, and people suffer with it for many different reasons: because of trauma, genetic circumstances, undiagnosed health issues, stress, and external circumstances. Sometimes it's a result of our own personal failures we're trying to keep hidden from the world. Many things can cause mental illness.

One of the great frustrations concerning mental illness is that we can't see it or touch it. A doctor can't show it to us on an MRI, on a CAT scan, or with a blood test. Of course, some symptoms can be seen, but we can't see mental illness itself. And that makes it even more frustrating for people who are fighting and struggling against it. So obviously, there's no three-step formula, no simple answer, not even a Band-Aid.

That's why I can't give you a one-size-fits-all solution. And even as a passionate believer in Jesus Christ, I want to respect the force of mental illness. Like the enemy, it has the power to steal and kill and destroy.

I also want to say this: If you haven't been through trauma, grief, or mental illness, you can't fully understand it. That's not a knock on you; it's just a reality that you've got to step into. If you haven't had suicidal thoughts, you can't fully understand them either. I had suicidal thoughts at age sixteen, but they left fairly quickly after I gave my life to Jesus. He saved me at the perfect time. So even I don't fully understand what that battle looks like. And those of us who've been through anxiety or depression don't even fully understand what we've been through.

But not understanding doesn't give us an out to be silent. We need to stand up and speak up. And throughout this book, we're shining a light into the darkness, even a darkness we don't fully understand. That's because we do understand Jesus—the Light in the darkness.

Depression does its best work in the dark. And I believe that depression and the power of suicidal thoughts gain their power there. Scientists say more suicides occur in the window of midnight than at any other time of the day. Depression, anxiety, and suicidal thoughts strengthen in that dark night of hopelessness when we feel like we might never "see the light of day" again. For me personally, depression tightened its grip in the dead of night, in loneliness and isolation.

From Night to Light

The good news is that we all have an opportunity to step out of the night and into light, to step out of the isolation and into community where we can be honest about who we are and what we're struggling with. And in stepping into the light, change can come.

I am not a doctor. I am not an expert. I am not a psychologist or psychiatrist. But as I've already shared, I've been down in the pit of depression and anxiety. Only my family and closest friends knew how deep that pit really was, but now I want you to know as well.

I've been down in that place where lies begin to overtake you. I've been down in that place where you think you're never going to be yourself again. I had days when I lost control of the peace I'd once felt in my body. I've been down in that place where you think you're losing your mind. I'm not talking about the "lose my mind" we flippantly use in our given life circumstances, like, "Man, I lost my phone for thirty minutes, and I was losing my mind." Not that kind of losing your mind.

I mean the real kind of losing your mind, when you're, like, *I don't know what's happening to me right now. I'm not in full control of myself. Things are going on in my mind and physiologically in my body that I don't have control of. And I think I actually may be going crazy.*

I've been down in that place where hope seems extinguished, and if you've been there, you can relate to me, and I can relate to you. But I'm telling you—and I'll say it a thousand times—with the help of family, friends, therapy, Jesus, and the weapon of worship, I made it back to the land of the living. And by the grace of God, I'm standing strong today.

What I needed in those months wasn't someone giving me a shout-out like, "Don't worry, Jacob. You got this. You can do it!" That's not what I needed in the darkness, and it's not what I needed deep down in that pit. I needed someone to show up and say, "I've lived through what you're going through, and I'm here to tell about it." And God sent someone to me who had gone through exactly what I was going through and had lived to tell about it. I needed someone to show up and say, "You're not alone, and you're not the only one," because I didn't know the world of mental illness exists the way it does until I was mentally ill.

And then I realized how many people live with some form of mental illness. The National Institute of Mental Health reports that in 2020, 52.9 million people 18 years and older in the United States did so—nearly one in five. They also report that "young adults aged 18-25 years had the highest prevalence of AMI [Any Mental Illness] (30.6%)

compared to adults aged 26-49 years (25.3%) and aged 50 and older (14.5%).[4]

But if you don't know any of that and you're suffering, you probably think you're the only one going through what you're going through. And I'll tell you what else I needed. I needed someone to show up and say, "Hey, this is going to be a bumpy ride, but you're going to get through it and make it to the other side."

Ultimately, I needed a miracle from God. And ultimately, I got a miracle from God, and that's why I'm writing to you now.

Those six months of anxiety and depression were awful, and I never want to go through that level of depression again. But on the other hand, I'm so glad I'm standing here as a result of that journey, because I would probably never be offering this message without that experience. And I would never have such compassion for people who are struggling the way I did.

And so, if you're in that place, I'm not going to propose some simple solution, and I'm not here to shout, "Come on, you can do it!" I'm here to tell you you're not alone. And I'm here to tell you you're going to make it through this by the grace of God. I take depression seriously. I believe it's real and a killer, but it's not bigger than Jesus. It's not even close to being bigger than Jesus.

If you're in a panic right now, if you feel suffocated by thoughts of suicide, I want to tell you I personally know a handful of people who have faced this fight and overcome. And I want you to know this too: You're not crazy. There may be a boatload of crazy in it; there was some crazy in my battle as well. But you are not crazy. You are God's masterpiece, and He is greater than what you're facing.

Maybe you're thinking, *But you should see the symptoms I'm having. You should hear the thoughts I'm having. You should see what my body's doing.* Well, I've seen all that before, and that's why I say there is crazy in it, but again, you are not crazy. God created you, and you are His handiwork.

There's something else I want you to know. We're here. The Stay Here team is here. The church is here. But we need a few things to change. For you. For everyone.

Change for the Church, God's People

The church needs to talk about mental illness more. The church needs to talk about depression more. The church needs to talk about suicide more.

Most often, the church hasn't publicly talked about suicide. When someone took their own life, at their service, no one said that's how they died. I've been to services like that. No one mentioned the person had committed suicide except in hushed conversations in the hallway. We didn't want to talk about suicide. We didn't want to surface the reality of mental illness.

Or maybe a family member was in the psych ward and we just said, "Oh, she's in the hospital dealing with an illness right now." We never mentioned it was a mental hospital. Or maybe someone we loved was out of commission because of depression. We said, "Yeah, he's going through a tough season." But we didn't want to tell people, "He's curled up in a fetal position at the house, and he hasn't moved in weeks."

And saying, "I've been having anxiety attacks" sounds so much more acceptable to people than saying, "I've had a mental breakdown." When's the last time you heard someone say that? Not anytime recently, because that doesn't float in society as easily as, "I have panic attacks."

I think we've got to strip all the pretense away so we can talk about reality. I think the days of our not talking about mental illness and especially suicide have to be over. Honestly, we don't have a choice anymore. Suicide is one of the fastest-growing—if not *the* fastest-growing—killers of young people. It's increasing at an incredibly steady pace, especially among teens and people in their twenties.[5] It's predominantly a white problem as well, specifically a white male problem. Seven in ten people who take their life are white men.[6]

On average in the USA, about fifty thousand people take their own life annually. Around the globe, that number jumps to eight hundred thousand annually.[7] And as I said in the opening of this book, every forty seconds someone dies by suicide. It's not some problem way out there, either. It's in your hometown.

Just the other day I was preaching to more than four thousand teenagers at Gateway Student Conference in Dallas, Texas. At the end of my message, during the altar time, I said,

> I believe somebody here has already made a plan. I believe you've written it in your journal, and it's in your drawer in your bedroom right now. You've already made a specific plan to take your life on a specific day. And if that's

you, I need you to know that you're not the only person who's read that journal entry. Jesus has read every word, and He's here tonight. He wants to bring light into your darkness. He wants you to know that He loves you and is with you. And He is for you. You've got the power to step toward Jesus right now. I know it's a bold step, and it will take bravery with four thousand of us standing around, but if that's you, I invite you to please put up your hand and let me see it, because I want to pray for you in Jesus' name.

And I would say that, in the next second, more than a hundred hands went up. It took my breath away, but in that moment, I knew Jesus wanted to step into the conversation. He wants to step into the fight. He wants to step toward people who are thinking about giving up on it all.

After the event ended, a young woman named Nicole approached me to tell me her story. She said, "Jacob, on July 12, 2022, I was within minutes of taking my life, but to calm myself down, I decided to watch a few videos on TikTok. Your video was the first one that popped up on my For You page, and it saved my life." Nicole also encountered the love of Jesus that night at the conference, just months later, and now she's spreading hope to others who are in the same place of pain she was in.

Let me tell you, we're winning if we choose to talk about it. The culture is trying to speak to depression and suicide, but honestly, I don't think society can save the world. So the church can't afford to remain silent on the sidelines. We must speak up and talk about mental illness. And that's why we're talking about it now. Whether for you it's depression or crippling anxiety or suicidal thoughts, we're not going to hide in the darkness. We're going to point to Jesus, because He has triumphed over all.

I hope that by speaking up, we can destigmatize mental illness and even destigmatize the struggle with suicidal thoughts. And I believe the church will be able to get into the conversation in the way we need it to once we wake up and understand the grip of darkness and its power that people face every day. Again, we can't just push it aside. We can't just say to people, "Oh, you can get over that." We can't just give them a simple TED Talk or one-line answer. We've got to realize we're talking about a powerful force.

I just hope the church can get to a place where people don't feel like they have to hide what's going on in their world. I see a church that leans forward instead of reeling back at the sound of these confessions. I see a church where there's no stigma for experiencing mental illness, for struggling with anxiety, depression, and even suicidal thoughts.

But what's stopping us from being that church? Let me share six challenges I think the body of Christ has to overcome.

1. Making it hard to be honest

I'll tell you from my own experience, being depressed is a weight. But feeling like you can't be honest about where you are is a much heavier weight. The pressure to be "okay" is intense, and sometimes that pressure is greatest in the church. Why?

Well, it's simple. We're a faith community, and our faith is supposed to be stronger than all the trials in the world. Our story is one of victory. We sing hope-filled victory songs. So when you come through the door of a church and you're not walking in victory . . . and you sit in a pew drowning in the darkness and feel like you're losing your mind . . . and everybody's got their hands in the air with their journals out and they're all shouting "Amen!" to the preacher's message but you don't feel anything . . . that's a weight. Especially if the church puts you in a position where you don't feel like you can be honest.

Is it possible for the church to become a place where people are free to walk in and comfortably say, "I'm depressed," or "I'm on medication," or "I'm in a treatment facility," or "I've been struggling with thoughts of taking my own life"? I pray so.

2. Teaching that suicide is an unpardonable sin

Does this surprise you? Well, enough Christian leaders teach that suicide is an unpardonable sin for this to be a huge concern. Talk about a stigma. But Scripture doesn't teach that suicide is an unpardonable sin. It clearly claims that only one sin is unpardonable—blasphemy against the Holy Spirit (Matthew 12:31)—but we don't have time to cover that, as it's a completely different subject.

So I don't believe suicide is an unpardonable sin according to Scripture, but I do believe suicide in the context of Scripture is a sin. It's a slap in the face to the belief that we are created by and for God's glory. Because when you choose to end your life, you cannot glorify God in that way.

No, you glorify God by staying in it and leaning on Him to bring you through one more day, one more night. That's how God gets glory in our lives. And we were created by and for His glory.

We all sin and come short of the glory of God (Romans 3:23), but I believe that for the believer, suicide is under the blood of Jesus. Yes, even suicide—"Where sin increased, grace increased all the more" (Romans 5:20 NIV). So though suicide is a sin, and a terrible one at that, it is a sin that's forgivable. Some people who take their own lives really do love Jesus, but they're sick, their mind isn't functioning properly, and the mental illness of depression is what takes them.

3. *Not offering the time and space necessary for healing*

Not everyone is instantly healed when there's an opportunity for healing. Sometimes it's a process, and we've got to give people time and space for it.

Now, can Jesus do a miracle right here, right now? One hundred percent yes. But at the same time, we need to understand that sometimes the miracle takes a moment. It's not immediate. The miracle may be that you make it until tomorrow, or you made it through the weekend to Monday, not that sudden—instantaneous—relief from all pain. If that's where you are right now, just fighting to make it through the day, it's okay to not be okay, and Jesus will reassure you that you don't have to stay that way.

I also believe the church needs to help us all realize and understand that God might not take all the pain away on this earth. Maybe you don't need to ask Him to remove you from the storm but instead to be with you in the middle of it. On this earth, there will be pain, but the pain can have a glorious purpose. You're, like, *But you don't know what I've been through!* I don't, but I know what Jesus went through. And He can come alongside you and carry you and your pain one more day so He can use you and your pain to help unlock doors for prisoners and set captives free.

4. Questioning the value of seeking professional help

If you're a Christian, some say you should overcome your struggle with mental illness with God's help alone. Others struggle with questions related to getting help: *Should Christians be on medication? Should they be in counseling? Should they enter a treatment facility?* Well, I believe the message of the church needs to be clear, and it's not simply, "Pray more," or "Believe more," or "Have more faith," or "Get over it." I wish it was that simple, but the reality is it's not.

Because I believe the stigma of seeking and receiving help comes down when we get real about mental illness, I also believe the church needs to clearly say what I'm trying to communicate in this chapter: "It's okay to not be okay, but it's not okay to stay that way." Then say,

> So we won't let you stay that way. If you need help, please get help. If you need a doctor or a counselor, see one. They are gifts from God. They can be a part of God's plan. All plans that bring healing are God's plans for healing. Any healing that happens in a person's life ultimately must

be the result of God, because every good and perfect gift comes down from heaven from God the Father.

5. Choosing to hide personal weakness

When I came out of the darkness and back to life—when I realized I was finally making it out of that hole and back into my right mind—I could have chosen to close the door on that season and never talk about it again. Honestly, that's the choice I wanted to make, because vulnerability is hard.

But then I realized it's my job to steward my story of a miracle of God's grace so it can help someone else in desperate need of the same miracle. The worst thing we can do is get through it all and then act like we never did. That just creates more of the spirit of religion. The church has got to be honest, and the church has got to be real. And when we do that, again, the stigma dissolves. The last thing the world needs is a fake church.

And of course, lots of times we hide while we're struggling. As I said earlier, for a long time, only my family, close friends, and my counselor knew how deep my depression really was. But even if you're not part of a church right now—and especially if you're not sure where you are with Jesus—I want to be sure you know something about Jesus. Hiding doesn't work with Him. Fake doesn't work with Him. He sees right through the façade. He's not into veneer, and He's not fake. So it's when we're honest with where we are, who we are, what we are, and where we've come from, that we become candidates to experience the power of Almighty God.

If you say you're "all good," guess what. You'll never get a miracle from God. If you say, "Everything's okay," you'll never experience the transformation of the resurrection of Jesus. But Jesus is here with you right now, and He's here to heal, here to save. For believers, there's resurrection in our story. We have hope. We may not be okay right now, but we're not going to stay that way. Because even though we may not be okay—and we have to be upfront about that—Jesus is. Jesus is a victor with scars, and He overcame the grave.

6. Not understanding that Jesus gets it

Did you know that Jesus was tempted to give up and quit His rescue mission to save humanity? On the night He was betrayed, Jesus was praying in the garden of Gethsamane with the weight of the world pressing heavily upon His shoulders.

He was hours away from His crucifixion, and the Bible tells us that Jesus was battling so much stress that He was sweating drops of blood. Jesus turned to His disciples and said, "My soul is very sorrowful, even to death." He went a little farther and fell on His face, and prayed, saying, "My Father, if it be possible, let this cup pass from me; nevertheless, not as I will, but as you will" (Matthew 26:38-39).

In that dreadful and dark hour, Jesus had to make the most important decision of His life: Quit and give up His purpose, or keep going even though it hurt like hell.

Jesus chose the latter. He overcame the weight of death and chose to keep going. So, we can now believe that Jesus understands where we are. He's in our midst, alive from the dead, having come through the darkness and death, and He's okay. Therefore, you and I can say, *Even though I'm not okay, Jesus is okay, and I won't always stay this way. I'm not a hundred percent okay right now, but Jesus is always a hundred percent okay.* We can say, *I feel like I'm losing my mind, but Jesus isn't losing His.*

You Have More Power Than You Think

Our words are more powerful than you can imagine. You and I can participate in our own future by confessing what's true over our lives, because in large part, our words determine our destiny.

If you're saying to yourself all day long, *I'm not going to make it. I'm not going to make it. I don't think I'm going to make it. I don't think I'm going to make it,* guess what. You're upping your odds of not making it. And you're also mimicking the enemy, because your heavenly Father's not telling you that.

The weight is real. The depression is real. The situation is real. It's all real. But there's a counterweight to this reality, and it's just as real. You may be going through the hardest thing, the darkest night, the biggest trial—up against hell itself—but you will come through. Jesus is real, and He's okay. So finish what you're telling yourself about your own destiny. Complete those thoughts with hope. If you don't see it or don't believe it, you can still speak it, because Jesus is in fact alive from the dead and has overcome the darkness.

You say, *What difference will this make?* I'm telling you, confessing and bringing Jesus into the darkness allows in a little glimmer of light, crashing into the blackout of depression. And that one ray of light can bring you another day of life. I know this is true. I've been there. And I know that you can be broken down to your core and confess that Jesus is a healer at the same time. The two things don't have to be congruent in time and space to be real.

Circumstances never fully prove the faithfulness of God; you can't trust them to do that. Sometimes they're opposite to everything we've come to believe about God. But the cross does verify the faithfulness of God, and it stands in history as proof that He is good even in the darkest night. And you can believe that about God even when you're broken down in your weakest state. Both things can live together. And when you start confessing the reality of who God is, light comes in. Use the power of your words.

You're like, *I can't*. You're letting your circumstances define your life. You say,

> My depression is horrible. It's worse than it's ever been. My anxiety is so bad I can't even go out of the house. I don't even know if I'll come out of this. No one has been able to help me. Nobody's been able to solve this. Nobody's been able to diagnose this. Things haven't changed. It's been like this for a long time. I've never been this bad off. Nothing's changed in weeks. I can't see a future for me.

Why not go on, this time with hope?

But Jesus is still okay. He's still solid. He's still true. He's still got His right mind. He's still strong. He's still a healer. He still loves me. He still has a plan for me. Jesus is still as good as He's ever been since the day He gave His life for me on a cross. I believe it. I'm not going to die; I'm going to live. I'm not okay right now, but Jesus won't let me stay this way. And every time I say it, I'm bringing Jesus right into the darkness, right into the situation, right into the depression, right into the voice of the darkness that's saying *Take your life*. I'm saying I've got another voice. I'm not okay, but my God is okay. His name is Jesus, and He's going to pull me through this.

It's not a simple fix, and if you need help, get it. But while you're getting help, use the power of your own words to create a future you're going to live out.

I'm going to say what the psalmist said in Psalm 118:17: "I shall not die, but I shall live, and recount the deeds of the LORD." I will not die, but I will live. And I will declare what the Lord has done. I'll have a story to tell of the faithfulness of God in my life. I'm not going to close it up in a closet. I'm not going to hide it behind a Christian-church veneer. I'm going to tell the world that's where I was, but this is where I am. That's what I was, but God brought me through. I was so far down, but God lifted me from the pit and brought me out again.

Again, if you need help, get help. Because I encourage you to stay here. Stay for your family, stay for your friends, stay for the church. Stay for the world. We need you. You have a gift, and we need your gift. You have something to contribute to make this world a better place, and we need that. But ultimately, stay for more than your kids. Stay for more than your wife or husband. Stay for more than your job. Stay for God and His glory. Stay today so that you can bring glory to God. Don't leave. Stay here.

You have more power than the enemy wants to make you think you have. When I was severely depressed, sometimes I didn't think I had a shred of power. As I said earlier, I couldn't function. And the enemy made me believe I had no power. But when my story started turning around, I realized I did have power. I had power to praise God in the darkest place I'd ever been in. And when I did, I just shoved it right back in the face of the enemy. I don't say that with a puffed-up chest, because I still struggle with anxiety at times. But by the grace of God, I will make it. I will not die. I will live, and I will declare what the Lord has done.

You have the power. Romans 8 opens with no condemnation and ends with no separation, and in between, no condemnation and no separation. In all things, God works. He works in the psych ward. He works in the pit of depression. He works through thoughts of suicide. He works even when a family member has taken their life. Somehow, He still works even in that. In all things, God works. In between no condemnation and no separation, you're an adopted daughter or son of the Almighty God. And the Spirit of God inside you says, *Abba Father, I have a Dad who loves me. I have a God who cares for me. I have a King in heaven who calls me His beloved child.*

One more time, you've got more power than you think you do. I'm not asking you to do mental gymnastics. I'm just asking you to agree with God. My God loves you even when you're in this pit, and He's with you in it. If you lean hard on Jesus, you'll see another sunrise. If you take your pain to Him, He'll carry you through one more day. And He will triumph over it all, because He is greater.

Prayer

Jesus, help me overcome the intrusive thoughts that come my way. I believe you can set me free from self-hatred and self-harm. Please do it now. Surround me with your love and with loving people who can help me find healing. Thanks so much for staying with me in this battle. I know you will help me overcome this. In your name, amen.

For Reflection

1. Have you struggled with suicidal thoughts in the past? Who knows about that struggle? Is it time to share your experience?
2. Are you currently struggling with mental distress—anxiety, depression, or suicidal thoughts? If so, does anyone know? If you are, please reach out to a safe person now. Visit www.stayhere.live/live chat or dial 988 for immediate help from the National Suicide Prevention Lifeline.

4

How Free Do You Want to Be?

In Christian circles, we love to talk about the freedom we'll experience in heaven. We say, "Aren't you excited about going to heaven one day?" We have conversations about it all the time, and it's like every other Christian TikTok video is about when the rapture will happen. We're always guessing Jesus will return any minute now.

But what about our life here on earth? What is it supposed to look like? Is the Christian life just saying a prayer so we can get a ticket to heaven? Is that what Jesus died for? Just so we can get through life, struggle through life, before finally being free in heaven?

Or is there more?

I believe there is.

Let's go to the Word of God to see what Jesus has to say about the Christian life. In what we call the Lord's Prayer,

He gives us a clue about what God desires His children to be seeking while here on earth. He says,

> Pray then like this:
>> "Our Father in heaven,
>> hallowed be your name.
>> Your kingdom come,
>> your will be done,
>> on earth as it is in heaven."
>> Matthew 6:9–10

Heaven isn't just a destination. Did you know that? It's not just some random place in the sky. No, when Jesus says, "Your kingdom come, your will be done, on earth as it is in heaven," He's not asking us to pray that heaven itself will come to earth. He's telling us to pray that the reality and culture of heaven will overtake and overcome the reality and culture of this earth.

Yes, heaven is a real place, but we can also experience it here on earth. Everywhere Jesus went, He brought heaven with Him. That's why we see demons coming out of people. That's why we see the sick being healed everywhere Jesus went. That's why when He walked up to Lazarus's tomb and the people opened it, the guy was alive—because heaven was with Jesus.

So what does heaven look like? What does it sound like? What does it feel like? Well, from Scripture, we know there's no pain in heaven. No weeping. No sorrow. No grief. No trauma. No physical abuse. No left or right. No Democrat or Republican. No school shootings. No wars. No depression or anxiety or suicide.

What *is* in heaven, then? There's joy. Freedom. Healing. Worship like we never experienced on earth. Unity. Wholeness. Jesus is in heaven, and He's telling us to pray that what's above will come below. Whatever is in heaven needs to invade this earth, because the Christian life is so much more than praying a prayer to get to heaven. It should look like heaven on earth.

And if there's no anxiety or depression or suicidal thoughts in heaven, they don't have to rule our lives here on the earth.

The Man at the Pool

I want to talk more about someone who got a glimpse and touch of heaven, as told in the book of John, chapter 5. Let's read the story first, and then I'll explain its significance.

> Afterward Jesus returned to Jerusalem for one of the Jewish holy days. Inside the city, near the Sheep Gate, was the pool of Bethesda, with five covered porches. Crowds of sick people—blind, lame, or paralyzed—lay on the porches. One of the men lying there had been sick for thirty-eight years. When Jesus saw him and knew he had been ill for a long time, he asked him, "Would you like to get well?"
>
> "I can't, sir," the sick man said, "for I have no one to put me into the pool when the water bubbles up. Someone else always gets there ahead of me."
>
> Jesus told him, "Stand up, pick up your mat, and walk!"
>
> Instantly, the man was healed! He rolled up his sleeping mat and began walking! But this miracle happened on the Sabbath, so the Jewish leaders objected. They said

to the man who was cured, "You can't work on the Sabbath! The law doesn't allow you to carry that sleeping mat!"

But he replied, "The man who healed me told me, 'Pick up your mat and walk.'"

"Who said such a thing as that?" they demanded.

The man didn't know, for Jesus had disappeared into the crowd. But afterward Jesus found him in the Temple and told him, "Now you are well; so stop sinning, or something even worse may happen to you." Then the man went and told the Jewish leaders that it was Jesus who had healed him.

John 5:1–15 NLT

This is such a wild story to me that I've been stuck in it for at least a year now. I can't get over how crazy it is. This place Jesus walked up to, the pool of Bethesda, has been discovered by archaeologists, so we know exactly where it is in Jerusalem. And it was a pool right next to the Jewish temple.

So Jesus was walking with His disciples on the Sabbath, and they thought they were going to the temple. After all, Jesus was a holy man, a rabbi. Maybe He was going to preach a sermon there. That would be the predicable assumption, and it's probably what the disciples were thinking. But instead, Jesus took a left and walked to the pool of Bethesda.

Now, here's why this is so strange. Not only did He not go into the temple on the Sabbath, but the pool of Bethesda was not a holy place. It was a pagan place of worship with images of false gods all around its walls. And people believed in this myth or legend: If someone lay around the pool long enough and got into the pool fast enough when the water bubbled up and stirred, they just might get healed.

But here's the problem: The pool's promise was fake. A spring inside it caused the waters to bubble up and stir. There was no angel in the water. So these people sat there for years struggling with their addictions, struggling with their sickness, blindness, or paralysis, hoping to be healed. But no one was getting healed there. No one was tasting freedom.

I think it's wild that Jesus chooses to walk into this dark place. But isn't this who Jesus is? Isn't He the Savior and Shepherd who leaves the ninety-nine to go after the one? Isn't He the Savior who goes after the sick and not the healthy? This is who He is. And while on earth, He practiced what He preached.

So Jesus goes up to this man and asks a question I personally think would have gotten Him canceled if He was doing this today. It's not a very "compassionate" thing to ask. He says, "Hey, do you want to be healed?"

I can imagine the man thinking even before he spoke, *Excuse me. Me? Are you blind? Look at me. I can't walk, and no one cares about me. No one picks me up. No one puts me in this water. Get out of here with "Do you want to be healed?" Go talk to somebody else. How rude. How insensitive. You don't even know me. You don't even know my story.*

I think if Jesus did that today, we would create the hashtags #meanJesus, #notanempathJesus, and #uncompassionateJesus. Because this generation wants a Jesus who fits their mold. This generation is hoping for a Jesus who will go to a man like that and say,

> "Poor guy. You're so oppressed. I've noticed that no one ever puts you in that water. Can I lie with you here on this mat? I just want to affirm that you're such a victim. It's so sad. It's so tough, man. Do you want to just sit here and sing 'Kumbaya' until we die and go to heaven?
>
> "Because I'm chill like that. I'm Jesus. I'm just here to listen. It's fine. You know what we should do? We should make a TikTok video and get you viral. Let's create a hashtag and make this justice project about how nobody throws you in the water. I think it'll totally pop off. Let's set up a GoFundMe to raise money for that. How about it?"

Well, that's not what Jesus did. Instead, He said, "Hey, do you want to be healed?" But the man was so into his issue that he couldn't see the solution standing right in front of him. "What are you talking about?" he basically said.

We Are Not Our Issue

The Bible's full of people whose issue we know, but not their name. I wonder if God inspired this way of telling their stories to make a point about what we so often are when we're stuck on a mat—missing out on the identity He planned for us.

A woman is caught in adultery in John, chapter 8. We never know her name, but we sure do know her issue.

A man born blind is seen in John, chapter 9. We never know his name, but we sure do know his issue.

And in Mark, chapter 5, is a demon-possessed man. He's cutting himself. He's growling. He's screaming. He's hanging around tombs. We never know his name, but we sure do know his issue.

Some of the unidentified people in the Bible with issues were no doubt more comfortable sitting in them than others, although the unnamed woman with the debilitating flow of blood was so desperately uncomfortable that she bravely reached out to merely touch Jesus' hem. But our culture today makes monuments about our issues. We make hashtags and create movements about our issues. And I believe and I'm fearful that many of us are so comfortably into our issues that we're beginning to forget our names, to forget the identity God planned for us. All because we love to sit in our issues.

God is searching for those of you who've been all caught up in your issue. He's looking for those of you who've forgotten your name, the identity He planned for you. And He's searching for those of you who've been on a mat for years and feel like you'll never get up.

He wants you to know you are not your issue. You are a son or daughter of the Most High God. You are His prized possession. You are His treasure. He left heaven to get to you. You are not your past. But if you want to get up, it will mean taking responsibility. The man at the pool could have stayed there on the mat. He could have said, "You know what? I like my mat. I've been lying on this thing for thirty-eight years, and I like the way it feels and smells." (I'll let you imagine what that thing smelled like.)

So many of us do get comfortable in our cycle of sin. We get comfortable with our issue. We get comfortable in our addiction. We get comfortable with being a victim. But Jesus says, *It's okay to not be okay, but it's not okay to stay that way. I have come to heal you.* And Jesus didn't die for you two thousand years ago just for you to struggle through life until you can go to heaven and finally be free. If you're doing that, I'm here to break it to you: You're putting more faith in death than you are in the death and resurrection of Jesus Christ.

But death is not your savior. Jesus is your Savior, and He came to save you now. He came to heal you now. He came to deliver you now. But you've got to do your part. Jesus already said, "It is finished. It's done. Your sin, it's finished. Your depression, it's finished. All of it, done. I dealt with it. I bore it on my own body on the cross. But," He says, "you need to receive it. You need to walk in it. You need to believe that I did this for you." But, again, healing takes responsibility.

What's also so wild about this story is the Pharisees' response. When the man stands, picks up that mat, and walks, they say, "Hey, how dare you carry your mat on the Sabbath!" What were the Pharisees mad about? The mat.

I think it's so funny that Jesus told the man to pick it up. He could have said, "Leave the mat on the ground. Yes, it's the Sabbath, but just be healed. Be free. No one will ever know you were sick for thirty-eight years. Just go on and live a new life, buddy. Come on. It'll be great." No, Jesus wanted the man to pick up the mat on a Sabbath so the Pharisees would notice. Because when you get healed of something, then you have a story to tell, and that's what the man did after Jesus later explained who He was in the temple. "Jesus healed me," he told the Pharisees.

In Romans 1:16, Paul says, "I am not ashamed of the gospel, for it is the power of God for salvation to everyone who believes." And today, Jesus is calling every generation to be unashamed of Him, to be unashamed of their story. Your past, your disease—whatever it is—doesn't have to own you. You don't have to sit on that mat all your life.

What If We Stay on Our Mats?

Imagine that man's future if he'd never gotten up from that mat. I can imagine what mine would be like if I'd never gotten up from my mat. I'd been told the gospel so many times, I'd gone to so many church services, and I'd had so many opportunities to accept Jesus, but I denied Him over and over. I went on mission trips and then partied with my other friends the next week.

But if I had never risen from my mat, then my depression, my insomnia, my suicidal thoughts, my anxiety, my addictions, my lust would all have stayed with me. If I had chosen to let that mat own me, if I had continued to lie on that thing, I never would have married and had my three beautiful daughters I love so much.

And I never would have started a suicide prevention ministry where we've seen thousands of people set free from self-harm and suicidal thoughts. I know we will see Gen Z become suicide free. We're reaching people now in China, Norway, Australia—all over the world. We've even translated our suicide prevention training into Spanish. If I had stayed on my mat, I never would have done all that. I never would have started Stay Here with my family.

And if I hadn't gotten up from my mat, I never would have been able to preach the gospel to millions of people all over the world. Since 2020, God has used me to lead more than a hundred thousand people to Jesus Christ. I never would have done that.

Picking up your mat isn't just about you, and it's not just *for* you. You've got to pick it up for this generation. You've got a story to tell.

When I was seventeen, I was no longer comfortable on my mat. I was miserable. I'd been faking being a Christian only by name, and I wanted to stop hiding. I have a feeling a lot of you are like I was.

People thought I was a good Christian kid, but I was lying. I put on the smile at church, but in my bedroom, all alone, I was so hurting. I was so angry. I was so sad. I was struggling with crazy anxiety, crazy depression. I couldn't get suicidal thoughts out of my mind. Anytime I got into my Jeep, I heard these voices in my head saying, "Just drive through that red light and see what happens. Just drive onto that oncoming traffic and see what happens. No one will even care. Just do it. You know life's hard." I was battling so many demons.

But then one night my dad took me to a men's Bible study. When I walked in, a seventy-year-old man with this glow about him, named Eldon Blanford, greeted me: "Well, nice to meet you." Next thing I know, I've dropped to my knees and started crying. Then I begin confessing my sins in front of my dad and all these men before the Bible study has even started.

I was so tired of being tired. I was so tired of lying on that mat. I was so tired of living a fake Christian life. I wanted freedom, and that's what I saw in Eldon, this much older man. I saw Jesus inside of him. He started to preach the gospel and talk about Jesus' forgiveness. And before he even ended his sermon, I raised my hand and said, "Can you just set me free? I don't even know what that looks like. I don't even know what I'm talking about. But I want freedom. Whatever my dad is experiencing, I want, I need. Can you do that to me?"

Eldon got up from his plush leather chair, put his hand on my shoulder, and said, "Lord, in the name of Jesus Christ . . ."

That's all I remember he said. As I've already shared, I'd been battling so many demons, and what happened to me then was crazy. I'd invited so much darkness into my life, but it all left me at the sound of Jesus' name.

I looked up, my eyes wide as I thought, *Oh my goodness. This is so amazing. I haven't felt this free in my entire life.*

Then Eldon said, "We're not finished, son. You've been emptied, but now you need to be filled with the Holy Spirit." So he put his hand on the same shoulder, and after I closed my eyes, he said, "Holy Spirit, touch him."

I opened my eyes when I felt something that seemed physical on my head. I thought, *Man, I think I'm in a cult. My dad took me to the wrong place. They're pouring honey on me.*

But no one was touching me. What I felt was the presence of Jesus, His hand resting on my head. And then

I began to be filled with His love, and all the pain from all the years of all my sins, all my addictions, and all the intrusive thoughts and sadness began to fade away. Each burden began to leave me, one by one, as the love of Jesus breathed in and breathed out, in and out.

I became a new creation in Christ Jesus that night. And more than a dozen years later, I'm still wildly in love with Him.

You can become a new creation in Christ Jesus too. But I'm not here to convince you to try Jesus, to try Him out. Because if I can convince you to follow Him with pretty words, then someone years from now might be able to convince you to stop following Him with more pretty words. You might watch a video or movie declaring Jesus isn't real, and it could convince you to stop believing in Him. No, I'm here to reveal to you that Jesus is real.

A Mind Full of Misinformation

Let's consider some of the lies we tell ourselves that might be keeping people—maybe even you—from seeking the transformation and healing Jesus offers.

Lie: Jesus will never reach out to me.

Another wild thing about Jesus at this pool is that we don't know anything about the other people there that day. The Bible says the place was full of the sick, paralyzed, and lame, but it doesn't say whether Jesus healed anyone else. If He didn't, I wonder if that's because they assumed He saw something in the man He didn't see in them.

Maybe you feel like Jesus will never reach out to you. You're, like, *Jesus loves only the people up at the altar jumping up and down in worship.* Or, *Jesus comes only for the people who do their daily devotions and pray an hour a day.*

But just like that man at the pool, I wasn't crying out to God, I wasn't in the temple, and I wasn't fasting and praying. He wasn't trying to change, and neither was I. We were both lying on a mat. I wasn't seeking God when I got freedom; I was sinning every day. I didn't want anything to do with God. But God came to me, and I'm telling you, Jesus is here for you. He even runs after us, and this is the difference between Christianity and every other religion.

In all the other religions, the god wants you to climb up a ladder to get to him, but in Christianity, our God came down the ladder to get to us. In all the other religions, we need to clean the house, set the table, and prepare a nice dinner for the god, but in Christianity, Jesus sets the table for us. He reaches out to everyone with the same invitation for salvation and healing.

Lie: My issue is too big for God.

I don't know how long you've been sitting on your mat, but I'm here to tell it's not greater than the blood of Jesus Christ. What He did for you is so much greater than what happened to you. Of course, when you meet Jesus and He heals you, it doesn't take away what happened to you. The blood of Jesus doesn't give you amnesia. And I'm not discrediting—nor is Jesus discrediting—the terrible abuse and trauma you may have gone through.

All I'm saying is this: Remember what Jesus has been through for you, because He knew exactly what you would go through and took it on the cross for you. There is healing for the oppressed. There's deliverance for the brokenhearted and the shattered mind. There's freedom for you.

Lie: I'm too much of a sinner.

I love how the Pharisees tried to convince the man to drop the mat and go back to the pool, but he was so emboldened by Jesus. They tried to put shame back on him, but he'd just been delivered from shame.

That's so like the devil. The enemy will always attempt to make you forget about the goodness of God. But the good news is this: You can come to Jesus a thousand times with all your messes and mistakes, and He will forgive you every single time. Jesus is a better forgiver than you are a sinner.

Do you think Jesus is shaking right now as He thinks about your life, saying to God, "Father, I'm so worried they're not going to make it. I've been trying to get to them, but . . ."? No, Jesus is confident about your future. But you need to choose to stand, pick up your mat, and walk forward with Him. He's already done everything He needed to do. He's already paid the price. He's already canceled your debt. He died for every single mistake you'd make.

Maybe you've been a Christian for a while, and you've messed up so many times that you're, like, *Man, am I even saved? I thought if I was saved, I would be free by now. I'm just a filthy sinner.* But after you accept Christ, God calls you a saint. He calls you a new creation. He calls you a son or a daughter. He's known all your sin but chooses to call you by your name. It's the devil who knows your name but calls you by your sin.

Are You Ready to Be Healed?

A few months ago I was preaching to about five hundred at a youth conference in North Carolina. During my message, I heard the Lord whisper that He wanted to heal someone's left pinky finger. As I finished my message, I said, "We all love altar calls, but you know what? Sometimes we don't get to see the miracle in the altar call. It's just packed with people. I want to demonstrate how real God is. I want to demonstrate that right here in front of all you guys. Does someone here have a broken pinky finger on your left hand?"

This guy in the back row said, "That's me, sir. That's me."

His name was Jacob too, and he was huge at sixteen years old. And as I got off this stage, I said to him, "I want to pray for you right now in front of everybody, because I'm not the healer; Jesus is. And I'm going to give Him an opportunity to be who He is."

Then, as I was walking toward Jacob, I heard another whisper from God, and I felt like Jesus wanted me to share it with everybody. Usually, I would never do something like this, but I said, "Jacob, did you break that pinky finger when you punched a wall?"

He said, "How did you know that?"

"I just saw a picture of you angrily punching a wall."

"Yeah, I punched the wall in my bedroom. That's how I broke my finger."

Then he began to tremble, and I said, "Jacob, God wants you to know He's going to heal that finger, and He forgives you for punching that wall. He knows exactly why you punched it, and He's not just going to heal your pinky but heal the situation you're in as well."

And then I said to everyone, "Keep your eyes open. Let's watch the Lord move."

Man, Jacob's pinky was wrapped around his ring finger, so messed up, black and bruised and swollen. His whole hand was fat from this break. I prayed for him right there, and after I'd prayed and proclaimed the name of Jesus for no more than thirty seconds, Jacob opened his hand, intently looked at it, and then closed it. He was overcome with the love of God as the Lord miraculously healed him in front of five hundred people. He hugged me, and then we cried together.

God moved so powerfully that night. And I believe He can heal you too. He can heal your scars, and He can heal your heart. He can set you free from years of trauma and pain. But you've got to be brave like Jacob was, brave to stand and say, "Yeah, I want to be healed. I want to be free."

I'm so tired of seeing believers just get through life. Jesus died for so much more than that. There's a prayer people used to say hundreds of years ago: *Jesus, I pray that you would receive the reward of your suffering.* And today I pray that Jesus will get what He died for—for you to come home. He died for you to have a name, to have the identity He planned for you, to be free. So how free do you want to be? Because the King is here with you, ready to show you just how good He really is.

Are you tired? Have you lost hope? Are you worried about tomorrow? God can set you free. Again, how free do you want to be? Because I believe if the other people there—all the paralyzed, sick, blind, and lame—saw what Jesus did for that man and had asked for healing, He wouldn't have denied them healing. But we don't read about anyone going to Him and saying, "What about me?"

Have you asked Jesus to set you free? Or do you doubt that He wants to heal you? But He calls Himself *Jehovah Rapha*, "the Lord who heals." It's in His nature to heal you. I believe Jesus wants to heal you even more than you want to be healed. Jesus is faithful and good, and He will meet you in your pain.

I know it's been tough, but just for a moment, can you get your eyes off your issue and put them on the face of Jesus? When that lame man on the mat looked at Jesus, he was suddenly convinced that he could stand, pick up that mat, and walk. Just one look at Jesus and everything can change. God can heal trauma. He can take away your fear. The Bible says He promises to give you a sound mind, a peaceful mind: "God has not given us a spirit of fear, but of power and of love and of a sound mind" (2 Timothy 1:7 NKJV).

How would that feel, to wake up tomorrow with a sound mind? No more anxiety. No more worries. No more panic. No more intrusive thoughts. Remember reading the first two verses of the Lord's Prayer at the beginning of this chapter? You really can experience heaven on earth. You will have a sound mind in heaven, but through Jesus, you can just as easily have it now while you live here on earth—if you want to be healed and you're ready to stand, pick up your mat, and walk in freedom.

Prayer

Jesus, I know you're asking me to stand and walk, and today I'm ready to do it. I've been sitting on this mat for too long, but now by the power of your Spirit, I'm getting up out of the pain, out of the mental mess, and into your arms. You can heal me, and I won't resist you. Please do it now. In your name, amen.

For Reflection

1. What is the mat you've been sitting on? How long have you been there?
2. What's holding you back from choosing to stand and walk today?
3. To what degree do you believe you can walk in freedom now instead of waiting to experience it heaven? Talk to God about this.

5

When Anxiety Attacks

Sometimes we think we're up against a battle or in a fight that humanity has never fought; there's no doubt that the research in front of us shows we have an increasing epidemic on our hands. But I remind you that this idea of anxiety is not new. In fact, in the 1800s, a great theologian and pastor named Charles Spurgeon said this:

> Quite involuntarily, unhappiness of mind, depression of spirit, and sorrow of heart will come upon you. You may be without any real reason for grief, and yet may become among the most unhappy of men.[1] . . . There is also a kind of mental darkness in which you are disturbed, perplexed, worried troubled—not, perhaps, about anything tangible.[2]

It comes as a surprise to many that a pastor like Charles Spurgeon had a lifelong battle with anxiety and depression.

His reputation as a beloved, powerful preacher; his joyful wit; and his manliness leads us to imagine there could never be a chink in his heavy armor. But many of us share the same lived experience. Being full of life in a fallen world must mean distress, and Spurgeon's life was very much full of both physical and mental pain.

> At the young age of twenty-two, as pastor of a large church and with twin babies at home to look after, he was preaching to thousands in the Surrey Gardens Music Hall when pranksters yelled "fire," starting a panic to exit the building which killed seven and left twenty-eight severely injured. His mind was never the same again. . . . His wife, Susannah, wrote, "My beloved's anguish was so deep and violent, that reason seemed to totter in her throne, and we sometimes feared that he would never preach again."[3]

That kind of inner turmoil Charles Spurgeon experienced produces anxiety, and this is not a new thing. This is an old thing that we must, in this day and age, battle with God's truth and some practical tools.

Anxiety has a cousin—panic. And both anxiety and panic are birthed from fear. Oftentimes when we talk about fear, we think it's always this evil thing. But if you pause and think about it, you'll realize that fear is one of the oldest safety mechanisms we have. We experience fear because fear helps us stay safe.

For instance, if you step into a street and then look left or right only to see a massive semi-truck coming your way, you step back onto the sidewalk as fast as you can. Your fear protected you.

A Sound Mind

An important part of your brain is called the prefrontal cortex, and it has skills that assist you 24/7. It helps you interpret data you've experienced, and then based on that data, it helps you predict what could take place in the future. Once you've had that experience with the semi-truck, your brain will say, *I've had some experience with this. Another semi could be coming. So I'll look left and right before stepping off the curb.* And if you see another semi or any other vehicle coming, your brain will say, *All right, I can't safely walk across the street until after this danger has passed.*

Here's where anxiety comes in: when your prefrontal cortex doesn't have enough information to predict a possible future, or it has skewed data, such as a traumatic event that took place in the past. This is why during the height of the COVID-19 pandemic we saw so much anxiety. And whether your drug of poison is CNN or FOX News, TikTok or Twitter, they all serve you information with an unpredictable future. Therefore, you become more and more anxious. And this is why science, medicine, and research can't solve all your problems.

We must come to God in faith, because faith begins where understanding ends. We need God's help in order to overcome that for which we have no data or skewed data. What does Scripture say about fear and anxiety? This is what Paul writes to young Timothy: "God has not given us a spirit of fear, but of power and of love and of a sound mind" (2 Timothy 1:7 NKJV).

You have not been given a sick mind; you've been given a sound mind. Sickness is not your destiny. Sickness is not your destination. Rather, God says, "I've given you power. I've given you strength. And I've given you a sound mind." You're going to need God's Word to get you through this storm.

I also want to remind you that you're not alone. Throughout the Scriptures, we see incredible men and women of God who dealt with anxiety and depression:

- Job cursed the day he was born and wished he'd been stillborn (Job 3:1, 11).
- Abraham called himself "dust from the ground" (Genesis 2:7).
- Jonah wanted to die when a worm ate his plant (Jonah 4:6–8).
- Elijah was the suicidal prophet. He literally asked God to kill him (1 Kings 19:4).
- And King David? One minute he's dancing before the ark (2 Samuel 6:14), and the next minute he's saying to God, "Why have you forsaken me?" (Psalm 22:1). This would be called high highs and low lows.
- Paul said he despaired of life (2 Corinthians 1:8). (We'll talk more about that in chapter 9.)
- Even Jesus, in the garden of Gethsemane, said, "My soul is overwhelmed with sorrow to the point of death" (Matthew 26:38 NIV).

If these men and women could be victorious in this life, if God brought them through, then He can do it for you.

Go on the Attack

I don't have enough information to predict the future, but I believe you can overcome anxiety with practical tools as well as with God's good words. So here are four tools to help you combat anxiety when it attacks you: name the trigger, shift the spotlight, stop catastrophizing, and add a comma.

1. Name the trigger.

A trigger is any stimulus—perhaps a sight, smell, or sound—that impacts our behavior. Do you know what suddenly creates an emotional reaction from you that produces anxiety? Maybe it's being in a particular place. Or a month or day of the year. Or hearing a song. (Some old songs are *good* triggers for me. Anytime I hear an old Frank Sinatra song, I rush to my wife so we can slow dance. It reminds me of our first dance at our wedding, to the song "Moon River.")

Maybe it's social media. Isn't it weird how we can be dealing with such anxiety and keep going back to the place that's depleting us? Social media can cause some serious triggers for many of us. It's not just about comparison. Maybe you've had a tough breakup in the physical, but you still follow that person in the digital world, and now you see them on your social feed happy without you.

Take the time to name the triggers in your life. This is so very, very important if you're going to attack anxiety, because so many of us don't even know what's causing it until we name it. As I've gone on a journey trying to grow and mature and get healthier physically, mentally, and even emotionally, I've had to go through this, and we could be here all day if I told you about all my triggers. But you can't solve what you don't know. You keep attacking all the symptoms, but you're not getting down to the root of it.

Now, this isn't just psychology; I believe that in the Bible, we see that Jesus went for the root of the matter time and time again. In the book of Mark, chapter 5, is this story of a man who is demon possessed. He can't control himself, throwing his body on the ground time and time again.

When Jesus approaches the man, in verse 9, He asks the demon, "What is your name?"

"My name is Legion, for we are many," it replies in the same verse, and Jesus cast them all out of the man.

It's a peculiar story, because then when the demons see a herd of about two thousand pigs, they say, "Let us enter them" (verse 12). They didn't want to be sent out of the country. Jesus lets them, and after the demons are in the pigs, the pigs run off a cliff and drown.

What I want you to see is that you need to name your trigger in order to change it. You have to name the thing that's causing your anxiety. It's not simply your environment but something you need to uproot to find healing, something you can bring out into the light. You have to name it to change it.

2. *Shift the spotlight.*

One thing I've learned over the years is that the way you view yourself, think about yourself, and talk about yourself makes all the difference in the world. One hundred percent of the time you will behave according to what you believe about yourself. And what you believe about yourself determines who you become in life.

For many people dealing with anxiety, it's birthed out of a place of shame. I bet you wouldn't talk about your worst enemy the way you talk about yourself. We do this to ourselves. We harbor negative thoughts. We talk negative ways. And so, because we believe we're less than, we behave like we're less than. Because we believe we don't deserve it, we behave like we don't deserve it. Because we believe we're broken, we behave like we're broken.

This is, once again, why we need God's Word: because God's Word is always greater than our feelings. God's Word speaks to us and declares that we are not our past, not our mistake, not even our future weakness. But we are a child of God.

An experiment was conducted with a group of people who had anorexia and a group that didn't:

> They asked 39 people (19 diagnosed with anorexia nervosa and 20 without) to walk around a room that included doorways of various sizes. The participants were distracted, asked to do a memory exercise while walking, not knowing that the actual experiment was to look at how they approached the openings. People without anorexia seemed to regularly begin to rotate themselves, to fit through the smaller doorways, when the width got down to just 25 percent wider than their shoulders. Meanwhile the people with anorexia started rotating when the openings were 40 percent wider than their shoulders.

[They concluded] from observing these approaches that people with anorexia use their perceptions of themselves in reconciling relationships to physical spaces not just consciously, but unconsciously. As they put it, "The disturbed experience of body size in anorexia nervosa is more pervasive than previously assumed."[4]

I wonder how many of us turn our position in life because we believe that for some reason we don't fit through certain doorways, even though we fit just fine. Do you ever notice that, when it comes to your weaknesses and challenges and issues, you somehow feel like there's this giant spotlight on you pointing them all out? Psychologists call this the spotlight effect. Our minds make something bigger than what it actually is.

For instance, we believe more people are watching us than are. This is why many of us walk through life with social anxiety. We might have a small pimple on our chin and then worry about it all day. More than one person has been quoted as saying something along the lines of, "You'll worry less about what people think of you when you realize how seldom they do."

See, psychologists tell us the spotlight effect is just . . .
False
Evidence
Appearing
Real.

The spotlight is not on you. You might have weaknesses, but you're not weak. You might have made mistakes, but you're not a mistake. You might have failed, but you're not a failure. Shift the spotlight. How you see yourself really matters. Many of us fall victim to what we believe others see about us, or what we think others think about us, or our mistake, or our failure, and it's causing anxiety due to a false reality. Shift the spotlight.

Let's go back to Peter, one of the disciples, who betrayed Jesus three times. It's fascinating that he denied Jesus to a servant, a little girl. She said to Peter, "You also are not one of this man's disciples, are you?" And he said, "I am not" (John 18:17). He was afraid, and this fear was now causing anxiety because he couldn't predict the future. In fact, the only thing he could predict was this: *They're about to kill the man I'm following, and now they're probably going to kill me, and the only way I can get out of it is by denying who I actually am.*

Peter denied Jesus while in front of a charcoal fire, surrounded by other people in the community. Then three chapters later, Jesus shows up. He's been to the cross and beaten death, hell, and the grave, and then He finds Peter out in a boat, fishing.

As I mentioned in chapter 2, Peter has quit as a disciple. But he hasn't quit life. He's stayed in the community, returning to his fishing boats, working with his brothers and friends. Judas made the same mistake Peter made—turning against Christ—but he isolated, which intensifies pain. And then what did he do? He committed suicide. Isolation intensifies pain, but being in community cures it.

When Peter and the others got out of the boat onto land, they saw a . . . What was it? A charcoal fire. With fish laid out on it and bread. Jesus said to them, "Bring some of the fish that you have just caught" (John 21:10). Jesus has created a charcoal fire, and now He's making breakfast, and it's from this place that He asks Peter not one time, not two times, but three different times, "Do you love me?"

Jesus is bringing Peter back to the trigger, the place of shame, and He's shifting the spotlight. He's putting Peter next to a new charcoal fire and giving him an opportunity for each time he betrayed Jesus. He's giving Peter that same number of times to confess and reconfirm his love for his Savior. Because Jesus was saying, "Peter, you betrayed me, but you are not a betrayer. And you failed me, but you are not a failure. And you made a mistake, but you are not a mistake."

Shift the spotlight. Turn your eyes off the issue and onto the solution.

3. Stop catastrophizing.

Catastrophizing is a way of thinking called a cognitive distortion. A person who catastrophizes usually imagines an unfavorable event and then decides that if this event does happen, the outcome will be a disaster. This is a psychological term for something many of us do.[5]

Have you done this? Maybe you're late to work, stuck in traffic. You didn't cause your situation, but now you're in it. What happens? You start catastrophizing:

> Oh, my goodness, this is it. I know it. I'm going to walk in, and my boss will look at me and say, "You're done." And everyone in the office will laugh at me and point and say, "You're fired." And I'll have to do a walk of shame with my

box and go home where my wife will learn I just got fired, to which she's going to say, "You are a loser. I'm out of here. And not only am I out of here, but I'm taking the kids. And not only am I taking the kids, but I met a new man, and he drives a Tesla, and he has abs."

This is catastrophizing. We make something out to be more than it really is. It's called a disaster dress rehearsal. And once again, why do we do it? As a safety mechanism, but it's an unhealthy safety mechanism. Many of us sabotage great opportunities and relationships this way. But when we catastrophize, we rob ourselves of the present moment we have to breathe and receive as a great gift from God. A thought attributed to more than one person and in more than one way often states, "I have had a lot of worries in my life, most of which have never happened."

Research shows that 80 percent of what worries us *will never happen*,[6] but you're behaving like they *are* happening, and you're missing out on the gift in front of you right now. We get only one imagination. How will you use it? To glorify your problem? Or to glorify a good God who has plans for you?

Let's go back to the prefrontal cortex. Did you know that it's what helps you enjoy music? It's why you dance, why you clap. It's your way of interpreting where the beat is going, where the rhythm is going. It helps you predict. I just wonder: Today, are you predicting a catastrophe, or life's beautiful melody? There's more to live for—a melody to your future. God has good plans for you. That doesn't mean you won't have to go through pain or suffering. But have you noticed that having suffered only makes you appreciate life more? Suffering gives way to beauty, to gratitude, to life.

Jesus said,

> Therefore I tell you, do not be anxious about your life, what you will eat or what you will drink, nor about your body, what you will put on. Is not life more than food, and the body more than clothing? Look at the birds of the air: they neither sow nor reap nor gather into barns, and yet your heavenly Father feeds them. Are you not of more value than they? And which of you by being anxious can add a single hour to his span of life? And why are you anxious about clothing? Consider the lilies of the field, how they grow: they neither toil nor spin, yet I tell you, even Solomon in all his glory was not arrayed like one of these. But if God so clothes the grass of the field, which today is alive and tomorrow is thrown into the oven, will he not much more clothe you, O you of little faith? Therefore do not be anxious, saying, "What shall we eat?" or "What shall we drink?" or "What shall we wear?" For the Gentiles seek after all these things, and your heavenly Father knows that you need them all. But seek first the kingdom of God and his righteousness, and all these things will be added to you.
>
> Therefore do not be anxious about tomorrow, for tomorrow will be anxious for itself. Sufficient for the day is its own trouble.
>
> Matthew 6:25–34

These are the words of Jesus—*Do not be anxious*. Your heavenly Father knows everything you need, so stop catastrophizing.

Name, shift, stop, and then . . .

4. Add a comma.

What should you do when your situation doesn't line up with your expectation? I'll tell you what you should do. Add a comma.

A lot of us think the sentence of our lives has been cemented by a period. We think it's over. We don't believe for a brighter future. We don't believe God for more. We don't even ask God to show up in our situation. We've given in to the darkness, given in to the pain, given in to the hurt, given in to the lies. There's no fight left inside us. But every one of us, as people of faith, have to see past the period. We even need to stop putting periods where God is putting commas.

I've discovered that a lot of anxiety has to do with concern about the future. But the comma is the mark of an unfinished sentence, and if you're breathing right now, you're an unfinished sentence.

There's this beautiful story in the book of Mark, chapter 6. When Jesus has finished feeding five thousand men (and even more women and children), He then puts His disciples in a boat on the Sea of Galilee and says, "Head on over to the other side." Then they row into a storm, they're terrified, and they're without Jesus because He stayed behind to pray.

Jesus leaves His place of prayer, walks out on the water, and meets the disciples in the middle of their storm. But before He shows up, we see that they are about to give up. They're drained. They don't have any fight left in them. Here's what's crazy: Theologians have realized that the

Sea of Galilee is only four miles wide, and the text says they'd rowed three to four miles. They'd nearly made it to their destination, yet the disciples were on the brink of giving up.

If you're on the brink of giving up, remind yourself to add a comma, because the other side is closer than you think. The other side is within your grasp.

You are an unfinished sentence. You've got to see beyond the false punctuation, that period you placed yourself. See beyond the circumstance. See beyond the season. See beyond the dark night. You might be saying, *I'm not healed*, or *I'm still not married*, or *I'm not sober*, or *I haven't found my calling*. But see, you're missing something. You're missing *yet*. You've got to add a comma and a *yet* to your sentence.

Your story isn't over, *yet*. The promise hasn't been fulfilled, *yet*. You haven't seen a revival, *yet*. Your business hasn't taken off, *yet*. Your marriage hasn't been restored, *yet*. Healing hasn't come, *yet*. But you can say, *Yet will I praise God. And yet will I worship Him. I'm fighting back with faith. God isn't finished with me yet.*

Prayer

Jesus, please put a comma on all the areas of my life where I've put a period. I believe that my story isn't over yet, and I'm putting control of my life back into your hands. I give you all my anxiety, worry, and fears. Please give me the faith to look at your face instead of my putting my focus on them. I know you're not worried about my life, so I choose to trust you. In your name, amen.

For Reflection

1. What is an area where you've given up? What do you think is God's plan for that part of your life?
2. Think about where you first let anxiety enter your life. Ask God to show you how you can begin to trust Him in similar situations.

6

Tired of Being Tired

If you don't like your life, give it to Jesus. He's got a new and better one for you. And if you're tired of striving to fix yourself, I've got great news about that too. There's a better way.

This chapter is a call to lay down your weapons, because you're fighting battles Jesus has already won for you. But first I'd love to share a vision I had from the Lord while I was praying.

I was trapped in a dark, spooky forest, wearing armor, fighting off wild wolves, bears, and beasts. The whole place was covered in spiderwebs. In the distance, I heard a voice saying, "Come up here!" I looked around and saw light shining through the trees and spiderwebs. I had little strength left, my armor was beaten and tattered, and there were holes in my shoes. I wondered if I could even make it to the light. But as I reached toward it, the angel of the Lord came through the trees and webs and rescued me. He lifted me into his arms and brought me to the arms of Jesus, who was standing at the bottom of a bright, regal staircase.

Jesus carried me up the stairs, and as we got closer to the top, all my armor began to fall off. I watched as it clinked and clanked down the long ivory staircase to the bottom. I heard the howling and growling of the beasts in the forest. They were angry that I had been rescued and released from their torment.

We reached the top of the stairs, and I saw the Father and the Holy Spirit sitting at a square wooden table with communion bread and wine in the center of it. I stood there, dirty and tired, wearing old long johns. Then the Lord spoke Zechariah chapter 3 to me, telling me I represented Jeshua in this vision:

> Then the angel showed me Jeshua the high priest standing before the angel of the LORD. The Accuser, Satan, was there at the angel's right hand, making accusations against Jeshua. And the LORD said to Satan, "I, the LORD, reject your accusations, Satan. Yes, the LORD, who has chosen Jerusalem, rebukes you. This man is like a burning stick that has been snatched from the fire."
>
> Jeshua's clothing was filthy as he stood there before the angel. So the angel said to the others standing there, "Take off his filthy clothes." And turning to Jeshua he said, "See, I have taken away your sins, and now I am giving you these fine new clothes."

Then I said, "They should also place a clean turban on his head." So they put a clean priestly turban on his head and dressed him in new clothes while the angel of the LORD stood by.

Then the angel of the LORD spoke very solemnly to Jeshua and said, "This is what the LORD of Heaven's Armies says: If you follow my ways and carefully serve me, then you will be given authority over my Temple and its courtyards. I will let you walk among these others standing here."

Zechariah 3:1–7 NLT

I was invited to sit with God the Father, God the Son, and God the Holy Spirit at the table. We held hands and gave thanks for the bread and wine. Then we ate together, and Jesus said to me, "This is all you need."

In this vision, God was trying to tell me I had been doing too much without Him. I'd been fighting battles alone. I got lost in the woods when I should have just sat at the table with Jesus. Sitting with Him is a sign of trust.

Do you trust that God has your best interests in mind? Or have you been putting matters into your own hands? God is calling us higher, to sit with Him away from the noise, away from what's making us so tired. Consider these Scriptures:

God, being rich in mercy, because of the great love with which he loved us, even when we were dead in our trespasses, made us alive together with Christ—by grace you have been saved—and raised us up with him and seated us with him in the heavenly places in Christ Jesus, so that in the coming ages he might show the immeasurable riches of his grace in kindness toward us in Christ Jesus.

Ephesians 2:4–7

You prepare a feast for me in the presence of my enemies. You honor me by anointing my head with oil. My cup overflows with blessings.

Psalm 23:5 NLT

The Pharisee and the Tax Collector

Let's read a parable from Jesus about two men I personally call "dead."

> [Jesus] told this parable to some who trusted in themselves that they were righteous, and treated others with contempt: "Two men went up into the temple to pray, one a Pharisee and the other a tax collector. The Pharisee, standing by himself, prayed thus: 'God, I thank you that I am not like other men, extortioners, unjust, adulterers, or even like this tax collector. I fast twice a week; I give tithes of all that I get.' But the tax collector, standing far off, would not even lift up his eyes to heaven, but beat his breast, saying, 'God, be merciful to me, a sinner!' I tell you, this man went down to his house justified, rather than the other. For everyone who exalts himself will be humbled, but the one who humbles himself will be exalted."
>
> Luke 18:9–14

Now, first I need to mention that this parable isn't just a simple lesson on the virtue of humility. There's much more to it than that. It's a message on the uselessness of religion—a comedic one based on the faulty idea that we can do anything at all to make ourselves right with God. It's about the madness of even trying. Therefore, it's a warning to let go of all religious, moral, and ethical stances when we're trying to take hold of our own justification before God.

This is, in short, a message and call to move on to the main point of the good news: Have faith alone in the God who raises the dead. So if you're feeling dead inside, this is for you.

Let's examine both men and the results of their individual approaches to life in Jesus' parable.

Two Men, Two Lives

First, forget about all the prejudice you may have against Pharisees, and give this one all the moral credit you can. After all, he's a good man. By our world's standards, he's a very good man. He's not a criminal, not lazy, not a misogynist. He doesn't take anything he hasn't earned, he's a generous giver, he's faithful to his wife and patient with his kids and consistent with his friends. He's nothing like the tax collector, who's the worst type of thief: a legal one.

The tax collector has the right to be a criminal for a living. He's a mafia-like man working with the Roman government, which allows him to collect hard-earned cash from his fellow Jews. The Romans have a challenging time finding certain Jews, but of course, the tax collector knows their whereabouts and speaks their language. He can take as much of the money he collects as he wants as long as he pays back the Roman government an agreed set fee. For years, he's been thriving off the work of his hard-working Jewish brothers and sisters, wealthy enough to own a Rolls-Royce and roll out with Off-White Jordan 1s.

And the Pharisee is not only a good man but a religious one. Not necessarily in a bad way either. His outward upright character is marked with inward discipline. I mean, who else is fasting twice a week and regularly giving 10 percent of their income to God? Any megachurch would give an arm and a leg to have a guy like that on their staff. To top it all off, he even thanks God for the happy life he has.

Now, remember, the author of this book of the Bible, Luke, tells us that Jesus spoke this story to people who trusted in their own righteousness. But Jesus shows us that this man comes to the temple to give glory to God. There's nothing wrong with that, right?

So what is Jesus trying to tell us about this good man who would be a proper candidate to take the role of head pastor at your local church? That he's in bad shape. But not *just* bad shape. This Pharisee is in a worse state than a rotten tax collector who just waltzes into the temple with no gift, no righteousness—just a small confession.

I know we would all accept the Pharisee into our church and even our home, but would you accept the man who has his hand in the offering basket to pay for expensive cars, shoes, and even prostitutes? Would it be enough for that man to come into your church on a Sunday, stare at the floor, and say, "God, I'm a sinner. Will you please be merciful to me?" Maybe we're saying we would forgive him and have mercy on him, but really, would we? I'm not sure. That's up to you to decide, but according to this parable, God says He sure would.

Two Men, No Game

Let's look at this moment from God's point of view, with my taking a little creative license here.

God is sitting on His throne, never sleeping, never taking a break, busy holding all creation in place, thinking and speaking things into existence, patiently counting all the hairs on our heads, making sure the rooster crows each morning, causing the earth to revolve around the sun, and caring for the homeless and the widows—all while bringing peace and wisdom to generals in the Pentagon. And now, in walk these two men.

The Pharisee proudly walks right up to God, pulls up a chair to the King's table, and whips out a deck of playing cards. He opens the pack, bridges them, does a couple of slick card tricks, and then finally shuffles the deck. He hands it to God and says, "Go 'head. Cut. I'm right in the middle of a winning streak."

But God looks at the Pharisee with a disappointed smile, gently moves the deck away, and tells him, "Maybe not. Maybe your luck just ran out, son."

But the Pharisee is persistent. He picks up the deck and begins to deal God a three of fasting and prayer and a king of no adultery. But God says, "Hey, I don't think you understand. This isn't your game. I really don't want to take all your money here."

"Come on, God," says the Pharisee. "How about just one game of blackjack, or what about some Texas hold 'em? I've been really lucky with Texas hold 'em lately!"

At this point, God begins to look a bit annoyed and says, "Look, son. I really mean it. Don't play me—the odds will always be on my side. You'd be wise to be like the guy who came in here with you. He ditched his cards in the trash can on the way here. How about you both just take a drink on the house and then head back home?"

Have you caught what Jesus has been saying in this parable? He's saying that no matter how hard the Pharisee works or how good his life may look, he has no shot at winning the game of justification and perfection. He's no better off than the tax collector here. In fact, he's worse off. Both men are losers, but only the tax collector realizes this and is trusting God's offer of a drink on the house.

Both men are dead, and the only hope in this parable is in the God who can raise the dead!

But wait a second, you may be saying. *Can't we give the Pharisee a little bit of credit here for his godliness? Isn't there a little more life in him than in the sinful tax collector?* But if we believe that, we're making the same miscalculation this Pharisee did. Dead is dead, and death is death. The tax collector has discovered the good news. He's come to an absolute end of himself. He knows he's finished in this rat race and that only Jesus can deal with him at this point.

But the Pharisee, on the other hand, believes his sack full of good deeds will carry him through for the rest of his life. He may be right, and he'll be fine. But what about the length of eternity with God?

No Goodness Apart from Jesus

Let's suppose for a moment that you're even better than the Pharisee in this story. Let's assume you're not tempted to any sin except the sin of envy. And even there, you believe you will never fall into that trap for the remainder of your life here on earth. But are you sure you'll always be strong enough to say no to that sin? Maybe the only reason you've been able to conquer envy so far is that you've lacked the opportunity to fall into it. But is your selflessness so profound that you can positively tell me you will never find someone you're jealous of? Is your iron armor really that strong and mighty?

Have you ever believed yourself to be immune to a certain sin or vice only to later fall into it when the temptation was strong enough? This has happened many times for me personally. The man who resists the five-dollar offer sometimes gives in to a five-*million*-dollar one. The loyal friend who thinks she will never betray her friend may do it if she discovers her friend is about to betray *her*. The pastor who thinks he's immune to the corruption of power finds corruption easier as he gains power.

We have no goodness apart from Jesus (Psalm 16). When we think we can gain a life apart from Him, we deceive ourselves, and the empires of sand we build will soon crumble into nothingness. True life and true greatness come when we give God our dead works. Life comes when He raises us into it. Don't strive for it; sink into it.

In the parable of the Pharisee and the tax collector, Jesus is saying there is absolutely no amount of human goodness or effort good enough to pass His test, and therefore, God isn't willing to take a risk on us and our human trust in works. He won't take our clutter and baggage as we hold on to them into His kingdom. But He will certainly take the clean emptiness of our death and recycle it in the power of Jesus' resurrection.

The Pharisee is condemned because he takes a stand on a life God cannot use. God commends the tax collector because he gives God something He *can* use—a dead man. The tax collector sees the truth: His efforts are not necessary, because it's all about Christ's efforts on the cross. We lose sight of grace when we live under the reign of bookkeeping. As we keep score of our good works and religion, we lose Jesus in the process. We can gain Jesus only when we let go of ourselves. We must let go of our trust in self-redemption. It's miserable to keep count of what God is no longer counting.

The Pharisee was counting on himself, and the tax collector was counting on Jesus.

Step into Grace

Hopefully, by now you see my point and have concluded that the Pharisee is a fool. You're right. But if you've also concluded that he's a rare breed of fool, you're wrong. So many of us make the same mistake the Pharisee did, day by day. We love grace, but we're so quick to run back to our own attempts to fix ourselves, by ourselves. Let me prove it to you.

Let's say the tax collector doesn't quit his terrible job as a scheming tax collector, doesn't repay everyone for his wrongs—doesn't even join a local prayer group or Bible study. What if he does none of that? What if he goes home clean, justified by God, yet doesn't do one single thing to change his ways?

A week of the same wicked living passes, and he goes to the temple and asks the Lord for forgiveness again. I'm telling you, he will still come home justified, clean, and forgiven. But you don't like that, do you? You're offended by the unfairness of this. The sinful man got off free again! We want the tax collector to come back with the Pharisee's speech in his pocket: "God, I thank you that I am not like other men" (Luke 18:11).

This is hilarious. We want the tax collector to come to Jesus, bragging about the sudden life change for righteousness, as if this would impress God. What we miss here is that he was already loved by Jesus, regardless of the good or bad. He never confessed that his heart was in the right place; he confessed that he was dead.

And that's where new life comes in. Let us never become puffed up by our own selves. We long to establish our own identity by becoming approved in everyone's eyes. We spend our days tirelessly striving for acceptance, people pleasing from the moment we wake up until we lie down at night. From social media to the workplace, our lives are filled with score cards. Truthfully, we hate this parable from Jesus because it plainly reveals the truth of our condition. We're afraid of the tax collector's acceptance because we know exactly what it means: we'll never be free until we're completely dead to our efforts of justifying and fixing ourselves.

For most of us, the business of self-help is our entire life, and that's why we must lay it down. We will never experience the wonderful grace of Jesus until we let it go. Grace needs to be taken straight. If you add works to the equation, you no longer have grace.

Jesus came to raise the dead. He didn't come to make bad people good. He didn't come to improve the improvable. He came to make dead people live. As long as we live like the Pharisee, alive in our own eyes, we'll continue to resent the scandal of Jesus, the scandal of His grace. But only once we're able to admit, like the tax collector, that we're dead, will we be able to stop scoffing at grace.

Let's face it. This admittedly is a terrifying step to take. You will likely scream and cry and flail around before you take it, because it means cutting yourself out of life's great game. And it's the only game many of us know. Let me give you some comfort. Here are three things I've discovered in taking this step:

First, it's only one step!

Second, it's a step out of a lie, a step from fiction to fact.

And third, like I did, you will laugh so hard when you discover how easy it really was, how short the trip to Jesus and His grace is. You were already there.

We must realize that only true life can come through Him. Before I knew Him, I was dead on the inside, and because of that, my life produced death. I destroyed so many people and things all around me simply because His real and everlasting life wasn't yet flowing through my veins. I needed a touch of heaven. We all do. Before I let Jesus transform me, I was alive, but I wasn't truly living. I had a heartbeat, but my heart wasn't truly beating.

The first time I felt God's presence, at that men's Bible study I talked about in chapter 4, it felt like breathing for the first time. I felt free, and I knew I belonged. I came alive in His presence, and I've been living with purpose ever since.

Death is the doorway to resurrection—the only way to become born again. Die to yourself so you can finally live with Him. We are either dead or alive, there's no in-between. Life is a person. There's no true life apart from Jesus.

Consider His words:

> I am the resurrection and the life. Anyone who believes in me will live, even after dying.
>
> John 11:25 NLT

> If you try to hang on to your life, you will lose it. But if you give up your life for my sake and for the sake of the Good News, you will save it.
>
> Mark 8:35 NLT

Prayer

Jesus, I'm so tired of trying to do this on my own. Help me. Help me trust you completely. I can't save myself, and I can't fix all this mess. Come into my life—not just the good parts, but all of it—and rescue me. In your name, amen.

For Reflection

1. Do you currently attend a Bible-believing church with a healthy community? If not, what is your next step to find one and start attending?
2. How has this chapter changed the way you think about what God requires of you?

7

The Prison Cell of Anger

In his book *Forgive and Forget*, Lewis B. Smedes wrote, "To forgive is to set a prisoner free and discover that the prisoner was you."[1]

One of the greatest ties to depression and anxiety is unforgiveness. Someone hurt you, you're angry, and you can't seem to let it go. Or maybe you hate yourself because you hurt someone or let something tragic happen, and so you lock yourself away in a prison of pain. But if we can't forgive others and ourselves, we can't truly live. And only through Jesus can we truly forgive anyone.

Let's jump straight to the book of Matthew, chapter 18. I grew up reading this teaching from Jesus in my home and in small groups, and I taught it to my students when I was a high school Bible teacher. Yet I believe the Lord has recently shown me a deeper meaning in the heart of this passage.

Here's the context: Jesus is sitting with His disciples, explaining what His kingdom looks like, what greatness looks like, and how He has a heart to seek all who are lost. Then the topic of forgiveness comes up.

> If your brother sins against you, go and tell him his fault, between you and him alone. If he listens to you, you have gained your brother. But if he does not listen, take one or two others along with you, that every charge may be established by the evidence of two or three witnesses. If he refuses to listen to them, tell it to the church. And if he refuses to listen even to the church, let him be to you as a Gentile and a tax collector.
>
> Matthew 18:15–17

If you're familiar with today's church culture, you know too many Christians believe this is a three-strike rule. We're supposed to confront someone one-on-one, and if they don't change, we're to confront them in a small group. And if they still don't change, we're to confront them in a larger group. And if they don't change after that?

We're to kick them out! Get them out of here, cancel them on social media, and tell them we never want to see them again!

Just kidding. But I have heard this passage taught like this, and I'm sure some of you have as well, likely played out in person or on Twitter. But let's go back to the last two lines in verse 17 to see how we should really treat people who simply won't change: "If he refuses to listen to them, tell it to the church. And if he refuses to listen even to the church, *let him be to you as a Gentile and a tax collector*" (emphasis added).

Jesus never tells us to kick people out; He tells us to treat them like Gentiles and tax collectors. So how did Jesus treat Gentiles and tax collectors? Let's read about the calling of Matthew-Levi, who's not only the author of the book of Matthew in the Bible but was a former tax collector.

> [Jesus] went out again beside the sea, and all the crowd was coming to him, and he was teaching them. And as he passed by, he saw Levi the son of Alphaeus sitting at the tax booth, and he said to him, "Follow me." And he rose and followed him. And as he reclined at table in his house, many tax collectors and sinners were reclining with Jesus and his disciples, for there were many who followed him. And the scribes of the Pharisees, when they saw that he was eating with sinners and tax collectors, said to his disciples, "Why does he eat with tax collectors and sinners?" And when Jesus heard it, he said to them, "Those who are well have no need of a physician, but those who are sick. I came not to call the righteous, but sinners."
>
> Mark 2:13–17

Not one time in all four Gospels, which recount the life and ministry of Jesus, do we find Jesus excommunicating a Gentile or tax collector. Instead, we sure can find many times when Jesus seeks out and loves Gentiles and tax collectors.

So here's the moral of the story: If your brother or sister still doesn't change after multiple confrontations, you're supposed to treat them the same way Jesus treated Gentiles and tax collectors. That means giving them even more grace than you might give a fellow Christian. It means not giving up on them. To keep pursuing them. Instead of judging and correcting, to try loving and listening. To not kick them out but bring them in. They may be spiritually dead, but love can bring them back to life.

Seventy Times Seven

The funny thing about this passage is that even after what Jesus said, Peter still seemed to think there must be a limit to how many times we should forgive: "'Lord, how often should I forgive someone who sins against me? Seven times?' 'No, not seven times,' Jesus replied, 'but seventy times seven!'" (Matthew 18:21–22 NLT).

Peter probably thought, *Seven is the number of completion, so it must be the limit to my forgiveness.* But Jesus said seventy *times* seven, which has two powerful meanings in the Bible—one not so good—that have nothing to do with a math equation.

Meaning #1: Vengeance

To better grasp this first meaning, let's examine a similar phrase in Scripture. In this passage, "seventy-sevenfold" comes out of the mouth of an angry and strong man named Lamech: "Lamech said to his wives: 'Adah and Zillah, hear my voice; you wives of Lamech, listen to what I say: I have killed a man for wounding me, a young man for striking me. If Cain's revenge is sevenfold, then Lamech's is seventy-sevenfold'" (Genesis 4:23–24).

Lamech is increasing the vengeance of the Lord to anyone who hurts him. This is like the ultimate revenge. This man had some anger issues. For reference, here's what the Lord replied when Cain said he was afraid he'd be killed as he wandered the earth, his punishment from God for killing his brother, Abel: "'Not so! If anyone kills Cain, vengeance shall be taken on him sevenfold'" (Genesis 4:15).

Lamech really put some heat on the Lord's vengeance, and it would be a good idea to avoid that guy at all costs!

Meaning #2: Forgiveness

Now let's jump back to Matthew, chapter 18, where Jesus mentions seventy times seven. He's saying your forgiveness should be the polar opposite of the anger in Lamech's heart. Lamech had a heart of vengeance, but Jesus had a heart of reconciliation and redemption. Lamech wanted to bind people, but Jesus sought to release them from their burdens and shame.

The second meaning of seventy times seven, then—forgiveness—is incredible. The Hebrew culture is fascinated with numerology, and nearly every number has a meaning. I have the number 555 tattooed on my wrist, which mean perfect and infinite grace. In Hebrew, the number 490—the sum of seventy times seven—means infinitely perfect; complete. Jesus is asking us to have complete forgiveness, perfect forgiveness, infinite forgiveness for the people who sin against us.

This passage of Scripture, then, is not about numbers or limits. It's about the heart. Jesus wants our hearts to be full and complete with infinite forgiveness.

The King and the Servant

If we still don't get it, that's okay. Jesus tells us one more story in Matthew 18 to further illustrate His point about complete and infinite forgiveness. This is a parable about a king and his servant who owed the king an amount of money so high it was impossible for him to repay.

I'll let Jesus tell you the rest of the story:

> And since he could not pay, his master ordered him to be sold, with his wife and children and all that he had, and payment to be made. So the servant fell on his knees, imploring him, "Have patience with me, and I will pay you everything." And out of pity for him, the master of that servant released him and forgave him the debt.
>
> Matthew 18:25–27

Amazing, right? What a gracious king! Unfortunately, this is not the end of the story, as the king's gracious heart didn't rub off on his servant who'd been forgiven the impossible debt.

> But when that same servant went out, he found one of his fellow servants who owed him a hundred denarii, and seizing him, he began to choke him, saying, "Pay what you owe." So his fellow servant fell down and pleaded with him, "Have patience with me, and I will pay you." He refused and went and put him in prison until he should pay the debt. When his fellow servants saw what had taken place, they were greatly distressed, and they went and reported to their master all that had taken place.

> Then his master summoned him and said to him, "You wicked servant! I forgave you all that debt because you pleaded with me. And should not you have had mercy on your fellow servant, as I had mercy on you?" And in anger his master delivered him to the jailers, until he should pay all his debt. So also my heavenly Father will do to every one of you, if you do not forgive your brother from your heart.
>
> Matthew 18:28–35

The servant didn't get it. Like Peter—and like many of us—he thought forgiveness is all about numbers and keeping score. But that's not the way of Jesus. In forgiving the servant, the king in this parable ultimately decided to lay down a life of bookkeeping and remembering the faults of the servant's past. As the apostle Paul states in 1 Corinthians 13:5 (NIV), true love "keeps no record of wrongs," and that's exactly what this king was doing—like Jesus, our King, does for us. Jesus did not come to keep score. He came to settle the score when He died on the cross, laying down the gavel of judgment once and for all.

We'll end up like this servant if we choose to live a life of keeping score. That way of living is hell on earth. Our job is not to judge others; it's to love them unconditionally, just as Jesus has completely and infinitely loved us and forgiven us all. By choosing a life of unforgiveness, we're throwing ourselves in a prison of hurt and torment. When we don't forgive, we hurt ourselves more than the person we choose not to forgive.

No matter how many times someone has wronged you, Jesus' command remains the same: love your neighbor as yourself. Forgive them. This may seem like an impossible task—and let me tell you the truth, it will be impossible if you don't have Jesus living inside your heart. Unforgiveness is like a cancer, and I don't want any of you to go on living that way.

Let's stop and take a deep breath. We've all been hurt, and I'm sure we've all hurt others. So let's invite Jesus in to help us forgive and ask others for forgiveness.

The Link Between Emotional and Physical Health

Here's one last story to help you find the courage to forgive. A few years ago, I was preaching on a Sunday morning at a church in Gig Harbor, Washington. At the end of my message, I walked off the stage to pray with people at the altar. One woman came up to me and asked if I could pray for her hands to be healed from rheumatoid arthritis.

I'm going to be real—her hands looked terrible. They were purple and stuck in a claw-like pose. I prayed for her immediately, but nothing happened. I felt like I was supposed to ask her how long she'd had this disease, so I did. She told me this had been the condition of her hands for two years.

I followed up with a second question: "Did anything traumatic happen to you two years ago?" Her response was so intense. Anger filled her eyes as she told me her daughter had run away with a boy two years earlier. She said she hated them both and hated herself for letting it happen.

After hearing this and seeing the deep-rooted anger inside of her, I said, "God wants to heal your heart before

He heals your hands, and I think you're so sick with anger and rage that it's making your body sick along with it. If you want real healing, you need to forgive your daughter, the boy, and then yourself. Forgiveness doesn't mean what they did was okay; it just means you're removing the noose from their necks and allowing God to take control of the situation. It's time to let go and pray for them instead of projecting pain on them."

She agreed and prayed with tears filling her eyes. After she'd finished forgiving everyone, including herself, she looked down, and I promise I'm not making this up. Her hands were completely healed. She came to the altar to find physical healing, but God healed the pain and anger in her heart as well. Even doctors agree there's a link between our emotional and physical health.[2] This miracle was a huge eye-opener for me on the importance of forgiveness.

So if you're ready to forgive like this woman did, pray.

Prayer

Dear Jesus, please come and fill my heart with your love. There's no way I can do this without you. Only you have enough infinite love to forgive me for all the things I've done to you and to help me forgive the people who have wronged me. I need you to help me lay down a life of bookkeeping just like you laid down your life on a cross and forgave the people who persecuted you and nailed you to that tree.

Today I'm asking you to help me forgive [fill in the blank], for the times they [fill in the blank]. I don't want to hold this against them anymore, and I want to love them just like you still love me. Please heal me from the wounds that have hurt my heart. I don't want to do this to others, so please give me courage to forgive those I've hurt in the past and to forgive myself for how I've wronged them. All my life I've lived like the world is keeping score. But today I'm choosing to live a different way. I'm choosing to live like you—forgiving and loving unconditionally. Thank you for being here with me. Without you, I could never do what I just did! In your name, amen.

If you prayed this prayer, you're moving in the right direction. You're walking in the footsteps of Jesus, with Jesus. But keep praying like this, because it's not a onetime thing. Let's live to forgive every day.

For Reflection

1. Were you able to forgive someone after reading this chapter? If not, what stands in the way of forgiving that person?
2. If you did forgive someone, how do you feel now? Or after forgiving yourself?
3. Who else do you need to forgive?

8

Stuck in the Loop of Stinking Thinking

Do you know you have nearly six thousand thoughts every day?[1] And many of those thoughts are conversations you have with yourself. You do talk to yourself, right? Everybody does. But what do you say? Is it all negative?

Here are examples of the kind of negative self-talk you might experience:

On your way to school or in a social situation, you say to yourself, *No one will notice your new outfit, and if they do, they'll make fun of it. You should just go back home.*

No matter how much you've accomplished, at the end of the day you say, *You didn't get everything done. What a failure.*

Dealing with money issues, you say, *You'll never figure this out. You'll always struggle with finances.*

Thinking about relationships, you say, *No one really cares about you. Why should they?*

And when you do something wrong, you say something like, *You're an idiot. You always mess up.*

And the negative talk goes on. Worse is when you say the same things to yourself over and over and over, stuck in a loop I call stinking thinking.

What you say to yourself matters more than you can imagine. The first part of Proverbs 4:23 (GNT) says, "Be careful how you think." Why? Because as the verse goes on to say, "your life is shaped by your thoughts." Psychologists call this the law of cognition. Essentially, this law says that what you think impacts what you believe, which impacts how you feel, which impacts what you do. Your life moves in the direction of your strongest and most frequent thought patterns.

You are the most influential person in your own life, because no one talks to you more than you do. I like that. But sadly, you may be talking yourself into a life you hate. That's why I want to help you learn how to end this negative loop. The world at large is becoming more and more negative, and chronic negativity has become an epidemic that's poisoning people's mental health left and right.

In many ways, negativity is a spiritual problem. But the good news is that by the power and grace of God, you can choose what you think about, and what you think about determines how you live. You're not a victim of your negative thoughts.

The apostle Paul said this in Romans 8:5: "Those who live according to the flesh have their minds set on what the flesh desires" (NIV). He wasn't talking about our skin. The word in the Greek for "flesh" is *sarks*, and it means "sinful nature." Essentially, he's saying those who live according to their sinful nature have their minds set on what the sinful nature wants to do.

What kind of impact does this have on us? Verse 6 in Romans 8 tells us, "The mind governed by the flesh is death" (NIV). It's darkness. It's destruction. "But," the verse finishes, "the mind governed by the Spirit is life and peace."

Think about it. The mind governed by the flesh is death. The news you consume, the TV shows you watch, the lyrics to the music you play over and over, the social media you consume that makes you feel left out or jealous or angry or less than, the people you spend your time around . . . they all create an inner script that helps direct your life.

If you find yourself feeling hurt, broken, or discouraged, could it be that your mind is set on the things of this world instead of on the things of God? Because when you set your mind on the things of God and the things of His Spirit, you'll find life and peace in all that you do.

Ways Negativity Can Play Out in Your Life

Let's look at some specific ways negativity can infect and affect us—if we let them.

Negativity bias

At negativity's root, we have what's called a negativity bias. Neuroscience shows us that negative experiences—traumatic, tragic, or at least unfortunate—imprint on our brains more quickly and stay longer than positive experiences do. They just seem to stick.

What do you think spreads faster on social media: something positive or something negative? The something negative. On any news app, which stories get more clicks: the negative ones or the positive ones? The negative ones. And have you ever posted something on social media that got a ton of positive feedback but one negative comment? Did you focus more on the positive comments or the lone negative one?

We can combat negative bias by being mindful of its existence and asking the Lord to help us overcome it.

Chronic negativity

Chronic negativity sends us into a constant state of fight or flight. God designed our brains to release cortisol into the blood system in any stressful situation. And that's a good thing at first. It makes us more alert. It makes us more focused. It makes us ready to deal with a problem.

It's good until it's not.

When we become chronically negative, when we're stuck in an ongoing negative loop, we always feel like we're in danger. We always feel like there's a threat. But remember, "The mind governed by the flesh is death, but the mind governed by the Spirit is life and peace" (Romans 8:6 NIV).

Negative neural pathways

When most of what you see online is negative, and most of what your friends say is negative, and most of what you say to yourself is negative, and most of what you hear about in the news is negative, all you're doing is focusing on the negative, and that creates negative neural pathways. And when you think a thought once, it's easier to think it again. Sticking around negativity can get you stuck in negativity. And very literally, negativity becomes a habit. It's a default mindset.

Your thoughts have incredible power over the direction of your life. They affect your relationships, values, and outlook. But the good news is that you have incredible power over your own thoughts, and you can change your direction.

Where You Might Be Most Prone to Negative Thinking

If you can't identify it, you can't defeat it, so let's identify what's holding you back from freedom and a sound mind, what type of negative thinking needs to be healed in your life. The four types below are outlined, among others, in various sources and with various terminology, including by the well-known Mayo Clinic.[2] But I tend to use these four, with these identifiers:

1. Relational cynicism

Cynicism is a general distrust of people and their motives. You can't trust people; you think they'll take advantage of you. *Everyone is out for themselves. Nobody's really here for me.* This type of cynicism is generally a reflection of how you feel about yourself. When you constantly distrust the motives of others, it often reveals that you don't really trust your own motives.

2. Negative filtering

This is finding the worst possible thing in any situation. It's overlooking what's good. It's overlooking what's right. It's maybe assuming the worst possible outcome. Simply, it's filtering out all the positive information about a specific situation and allowing in only the negative information, real or not.

Your friend is running late and you think, *Oh my gosh, she must have been in an accident,* but you thought that the last eighteen times she was late too. Or you go on vacation and ruminate only on what's wrong with it. Or you meet someone, and within the first ten minutes you've determined everything you think is wrong with them.

3. Absolutist thinking

This is all-or-nothing, black-and-white thinking. If a man hurts you, all men are bad. If a woman lies to you, all women are liars. This is an irrational belief system. For example, your using absolute words or phrases like *always, totally, never,* and *entire* instead of non-absolute words or phrases like *sometimes* or *it's likely* says you have a black-and-white view of the world. So if you say things like, "Rainy days are always depressing" instead of, "Sometimes rainy days are depressing," leaving out the possibility you could be happy on a rainy day, you may be stuck in the loop of absolutist thinking.

4. Blaming

This is simply believing that you're always a victim. Someone got in your way or took your opportunity or didn't give you a chance. You feel like you don't have any control over what's happening to you. You feel like you're a victim of circumstances, and the world has stacked the deck against you.

Reviewing these types of negative thinking raises this question: If you find yourself constantly jealous or critical, or discontent or assuming the worst, or negative about other people or hard on yourself, can you change? Can you shift from a chronically negative mindset to one that's full of faith and reflects the heart and character of Jesus? Can you shift?

The answer is yes you can. It may not be easy, but all things are possible with God.

How You Can Move from Death to Life

Let's look at one of the most powerful illustrations of the mind in the Old Testament. At the beginning of 1 Samuel 30, it was a bad day for King David—a really bad day: "When David and his men reached Ziklag, they found it destroyed by fire and their wives and sons and daughters taken captive. So David and his men wept aloud until they had no strength left to weep" (verses 3-4 NIV).

Have you ever wept aloud until you had no strength left to weep? For David, it got even worse. Continuing in the

NIV throughout this passage, "David was greatly distressed because the men were talking of stoning him; each one was bitter in spirit because of his sons and daughters" (verse 6). Yet in the middle of David's worst and lowest moment, the end of verse 6 tells us, "David found strength in the LORD his God."

If you too are living under an avalanche of negativity, whether or not it's come through any fault of your own, it's time for you to find some strength. Not in your own power, not in your own mere positive thinking (despite advice from the Mayo Clinic and elsewhere), but in the power of the life-changing presence of God and in the power of His Word.

In the King James Version, verse 6 reads, "David encouraged himself in the LORD his God." And in a world of chronic negativity, and in the middle of your darkest moments, you also need to learn to encourage yourself in the Lord. We don't know how David encouraged himself in the Lord in 1 Samuel 30, but we do know what two things he did in Psalm 103, and you can do the same.

1. Remember who God is and what He's done

Again turning to the NIV, we see in Psalm 103 that David is encouraging himself in the Lord when he remembers who God is and what He's done. He's saying, "Praise the LORD, my soul" (verse 1). Not, "Praise you, God." He's saying, *Hey, soul, praise the Lord.* He went on to say in that verse, "All my inmost being, praise his holy name." He's saying, *Self, start worshipping God. I know you're tired, but get up and praise him anyway.*

In verse 2 he says, "Praise the LORD, my soul, and forget not all his benefits." He's telling himself, *Don't forget who God is and what He's done.* And in verses 3 through 5, David says God is the one "who forgives all your sins and heals all your diseases, who redeems your life from the pit and crowns you with love and compassion, who satisfies your desires with good things."

David is getting encouraged here. *Hey, remember, David, God anointed you as king. He chose you. He set you apart. He delivered you from the lion and the bear. He gave you the faith and the courage to stand up to Goliath. Remember that He never leaves you, that He never forsakes you.*

In Psalm 103:8, he says something you may have heard before: "The LORD is compassionate and gracious, slow to anger, abounding in love" (NIV). This wasn't the only time David said these words about God. We find them in his Psalm 86 and Psalm 145. The Lord is compassionate. He's gracious. He's slow to anger. The Lord loves. He said it again and again.

And David wasn't the first one to use these words. He plagiarized God, but that was okay. God said them of Himself in Exodus 34:6: "The LORD, the LORD, the compassionate and gracious God, slow to anger, abounding in love and faithfulness" (NIV).

2. *Ruminate on God's Word*

What's interesting is that when things got bad, David didn't have to go searching for the Scripture he needed. He'd already hidden God's Word in his heart, and he said the same thing to himself over and over.

I want to give you a tool to help you encourage yourself: start acting like my goats, Harry, Chewy, and Jawa. I'm serious. Goats digest their food much differently than we do—it's called *ruminating*. They chew a mouthful of grass or leaves again and again, and then they swallow it before throwing it back up in their mouth to chew it again and swallow it again and throw it back up into their mouth again to chew it some more.

Why do goats do that? They want to get every bit of nutrition out of that grass. They ruminate. And the same Hebrew word in the Old Testament translated to *meditate* can also be translated to *ruminate*. Ruminate, meditate, chew, enjoy, get every bit of spiritual nutrition from God's Word over and over until it changes you. David found his verse to ruminate or meditate on—"The LORD is compassionate and gracious, slow to anger, abounding in love" (Psalm 103:8 NIV)—and with it he found strength and encouragement to make it through the darkest nights. And you need to find yours.

Earlier, we went over four types of negative thinking, and now I want to give you not four types of positive thinking but four powerful truths to ruminate on. To meditate on, to help get you out of the loop you're stuck in.

1. If you're battling **relational cynicism**, you can say over and over, *With God's help, I will get rid of all bitterness and skepticism. I choose to believe the best about others and be kind, compassionate, and loving. I will love and forgive others as Jesus has loved and forgiven me.*

2. If you're experiencing **negative filtering**, you can say, *By God's power, I take every thought captive and make it obedient to the truth of Christ. Because God is good, I choose to think on what's good, right, true, helpful, and worthy of praise. As I trust in the Lord, His peace will guard my heart, soul, and mind in Christ Jesus.*

3. If you find yourself lost in **absolutist thinking**, you can say, *As Jesus loved and accepted me, I will love and accept others. Rather than always being right, I'm called to always be loving. Rather than just making a point, I choose to make a difference. In humility, I choose to love others above myself.*

4. And if you're drawn to **blaming**, you can say, *God has given me a mind of my own. By His grace, I will own my choices and choose His best for me. I've been given everything I need to accomplish all God wants me to do. In Christ—by His power, by His blood, by His Spirit—I will overcome. I am an overcomer by the blood of the Lamb and by the words of this testimony.*

The mind governed by the flesh is death, destruction, darkness, and negativity. Who do you think that's from? Our spiritual enemy, the father of lies, who comes to steal, kill, and destroy. But again, Jesus said, "I've come to give you life and life to the full" (John 10:10, paraphrased). The mind governed by the flesh is death, but the mind governed by the Spirit is life and joy and peace.

So will you continue to be swept up by the latest gossip or bad news and bring yourself down to the lowest common denominator of popular opinion? Or will you stand up for something that brings glory to God? We're not victims of what goes on in the world. We can choose to see through God's lens. We can choose to look for the good in people. We can choose to be loving and kind and full of grace, because our thoughts have incredible power and we have incredible power over them. And therefore, we will not be conformed to the patterns of this world but instead be transformed. How? By allowing God to renew our minds and change the way we think (Romans 12:2).

If you're ready to break out of the loop of negative thinking, pray this prayer below and choose to draw a line in the sand. No more ruminating on the negatives. It's time to meditate on the Word of God.

Prayer

Jesus, I want freedom from the cycle of negativity I've found myself in. Today I'm asking you to give me new thought patterns and a new lens through which I see myself, my situation, and the world around me. To remember who you are and what you've done for me. Help me meditate on your Word, and let it produce fruit in my life that drowns out all the negative roots I've let grow around me. In your name I pray, amen.

For Reflection

1. What one Scripture verse can you start meditating on to combat negative thinking?
2. What is causing negative thinking for you right now? How can you cut that out of your life?

9

Jesus Can Heal Your Trauma

Now we'll talk about trauma, one of the most challenging of all the subjects we're covering in this book. It's a topic that, quite honestly, we may not hear about in churches frequently. But we should, because Jesus is not only familiar with trauma, but He can heal it.

It's likely that at some point in your life you've endured some kind of trauma, and so as I write this chapter, it's with real awareness that you may have been wounded through one or more horrible experiences and struggle daily with deep emotional pain. That's why I walk into this topic prayerfully and carefully. I've also been praying that as you read these pages, you'll begin to find the healing available to you through the love of Jesus.

I grew up in a generation that didn't necessarily take trauma seriously. We'd say, "Get over it. It can't be that bad." Or, "You're still sad? Wasn't that, like, six months ago?" Or, "Suck it up. Stop crying about it. Put some dirt on that wound and get back out there." But what I've grown to learn is that you can't just move past trauma; you have to heal from it. You don't get over it; you must go through it.

What Is Trauma?

It's possible to think trauma is only physical—like suffering a severe head trauma. But according to *Merriam-Webster Dictionary*, a trauma can be either "an injury" or "an emotional upset."[1] So while trauma can be physical, it can also be emotional. And that's why it's so important to remember that the wounds we can't see in a person can hurt as much as the ones we can see. And sometimes they take even longer to heal.

Perhaps someone hurt you and now you don't know how to trust people. Or you find it difficult to trust God. Maybe you grew up in poverty, and so you carry a dysfunctional fear of never having enough no matter how much money is in your bank account. Or you're so traumatized from something done to you that you worry someone will do the same thing to one of your children.

Emotional trauma comes in three types:

1. Acute trauma

Acute trauma is a response to a onetime event. Maybe you were in a horrible car accident or you survived a devastating natural disaster (Hurricane Ian, for example, which is striking Southern Florida as I'm writing this). It might have been a complicated birth or a miscarriage, losing your business or your senior year of high school due to COVID-19, or maybe you were sexually assaulted in college. It was a onetime event, it was horrible, and it was traumatic.

2. *Chronic trauma*

Chronic trauma is a response from prolonged or repeated events. For example, you may have been bullied all the way through junior high, or you've experienced racism for most of your life. Some of you were raised in a home with alcohol or drug abuse and you never felt safe. Others of you were sexually abused multiple times or repeatedly shown pornography—and by someone who should have been protecting you instead of harming you.

3. *Complex trauma*

Complex trauma is a response to multiple and ongoing events. This is when you see some combination of all the things we talked about above. There's chemical abuse, emotional abuse, physical abuse, sexual abuse—and the list could go on.

No matter what you've been through or at what level, trauma changes you, and it changes your perspective. It can change how you see people, it can change how you see God, and it can change your outlook on life.

I experienced emotional spiritual abuse from a pastor, and there was a time when I wondered if I would ever want to do ministry again. But after counseling, prayer, and healing through exposure to other pastors, here I am today, healed and free.

The Apostle Paul's Experience

Let's investigate the life of the apostle Paul, the person most of us would never think was traumatized, the guy who wrote two thirds of the New Testament, the man who said, "To live is Christ, and to die is gain" (Philippians 1:21).

Paul experienced all three types of emotional trauma—acute, chronic, and complex—and we can go all the way back to his conversion experience in Acts 9 to see how all that began. My conversion to Christ was a Hallmark Channel movie compared to his. On his way to arrest and kill more Christians—people he felt obligated to persecute—a light from heaven suddenly knocked him onto the ground. (The only light I know of that knocks people to the ground is lightning. Could Paul have been struck by lightning?)

And then a voice from heaven speaks. It doesn't say, "Hello, my special servant. I have chosen thou." No, the voice says, "Saul, why are you persecuting me?" (Acts 9:4). We know from Acts 13:9 that Paul was known by both Saul and Paul.

So God knocks him down and then confronts him, and he's blind for three days before he's healed after a man named Ananias prays for him. Then this Christian-killer becomes a killer Christian preacher. He preaches the gospel and sees countless lives saved.

For the rest of his life, Paul endured terrible hardship and abuse, oftentimes running for his life. In fact, in any town Paul went to preach, he eventually had to try to escape to avoid being killed. He was beaten, stoned, imprisoned, trafficked, and often homeless. He endured ongoing severe trauma, both physical and emotional. Yet Paul healed emotionally, and I want to show you how he found that healing in three steps—steps you can take as well.

Step 1: Paul acknowledged and processed his pain.

Maybe you're trying to put a trauma you've been through aside and act like it never happened. But you won't heal if you ignore the wound, you won't heal if you suppress the wound, and you won't heal if you try to forget the wound. You start to heal only when you both acknowledge and process it.

So first you have to admit what happened to you: "I was abused," or "I grew up in a dysfunctional family," or "I was cheated on," or "I was raped," or "I was abandoned." But we don't want to acknowledge our trauma because we feel vulnerable, helpless, like it's better to ignore what happened than to process it. But then instead of seeking connection, we prioritize protection. Instead of taking our pain to trusted people, we push them away. But we don't heal in isolation; we heal in communities. We're always better together. Scripture says when we confess our faults, our pain, and our trauma to one another, and we pray for one another, we may be healed (James 5:16).

If you ignore the pain, the wound will remain, and you'll go somewhere else to cope. You'll go to drugs, or to alcohol, or to sex, or to food as a coping mechanism. Or you'll go to what I often do—work. Many men become workaholics to stuff the pain away.

Paul both acknowledged and processed his trauma, and you can find him doing so several times in the Bible—

especially when he's telling what he's been through in 2 Corinthians 11, starting in verse 23. You can read the whole passage if you want, but right now I'll give you an overview.

He says he was in prison many times and beaten too many times to count. Five times he was beaten with thirty-nine lashes, not forty. (If you died after thirty-nine lashes, in court they'd say you died from a beating. But if you died from forty lashes, that would be murder.) Three times he was beaten with rods. He was stoned—with rocks, by the way, not marijuana. He was shipwrecked three times, he almost starved to death, and he nearly froze in the cold. He was in danger everywhere he went from, well, you name it. Robbers; his own people, the Jews; Gentiles; the city, the wilderness, the sea . . .

I need to pause to make sure you realize that if you've ever hurt so deeply that you didn't know if you wanted to go on, this guy who wrote two thirds of the New Testament was there too. In 2 Corinthians 1:8, Paul wrote about him and his companions, "We were under great pressure, far beyond our ability to endure, so that we *despaired of life itself*" (NIV, emphasis added).

We don't heal when we ignore our pain. We have to acknowledge it and process it. I encourage you to find the right safe place with the right safe people to process the pain of your trauma. Your trusted friends, your family, or your pastor. A Christian counselor who's trained to help.

Step 2: Paul pressed into God.

After acknowledging our trauma, we must prayerfully press into God with it. We take it to God, we cry out to

God, we talk to God, and we might even vent to God. In 2 Corinthians 12, this is what Paul said he did with what he called a thorn in his life. We don't know what it was (scholars have guessed all sorts of things), but we know it tormented him.

Paul wrote about this thorn, "Three times I pleaded with the Lord, that it should leave me" (verse 8). Most scholars say this was likely three seasons of ongoing prayer, not three single prayers. But notice that Paul didn't blame God for the thorn. Instead, he took it to God, and he prayed, and he pleaded, and he cried out for help.

It seems to me that almost everyone has a thorn—that something we wish we didn't have. But in the very same way Paul did, you can take your hurt to God, and you can take it to Him again, and you can take it to Him a third time, and you can unload on Him each time. You can say, *God, I don't understand. Why did this happen? Why did you let this happen when you could have stopped it?* You can be totally and completely honest with Him.

So don't hold back. God can handle it. Scripture talks about "casting all your cares on him, because he cares about you" (1 Peter 5:7 CSB). Your burdens aren't a burden to Him. Give Him the hurt from your heart and say, *God, please take it away.*

Of course, God might not take it away. He didn't remove Paul's thorn from his life. But Paul says the Lord told him, "My grace is sufficient for you, for my power is made perfect in weakness" (2 Corinthians 12:9). And then Paul gets it. He says in verse 10, "That is why, for Christ's sake, I delight in weaknesses, in insults, in hardships, in persecutions, in difficulties. For when I am weak, then I am strong" (NIV).

Strength like that comes only from the presence of God. Take your pain to Him, and even if He doesn't take it away, He says His grace is all you need.

Nothing can change your past, but God can heal your broken heart. The Bible tells us "the LORD is near to the brokenhearted and saves the crushed in spirit" (Psalm 34:18).

Step 3: Paul realized the purpose in his trauma.

Last, we must realize the purpose in our trauma. I'm a little hesitant to say this, because I know if you're hurting, you're thinking it's too soon. But after you acknowledge and process your pain and take it to God, you may say something similar to what Paul said even after being beaten, shipwrecked, stoned, and left for dead: "Praise be to the God and Father of our Lord Jesus Christ, the Father of compassion and the God of all comfort, who comforts us in all our troubles" (2 Corinthians 1:3–4 NIV).

Why does God comfort us? Because He loves us, yes, but also for this purpose Paul realized in the rest of verse 4: "So that we can comfort those in any trouble with the comfort we ourselves receive from God" (NIV).

I won't make this all about me, but I've gone through some intense, deep, and painful trauma. At times I was so afraid of losing myself in the dark pit of my own pain. But somehow God drew me out and helped me discover how the pain could be used. And we know what Romans 8:28 says: "In all things [even in our most painful and broken moments] God works for the good of those who love him, who have been called according to his purpose" (NIV).

When I was in the pit, I chose to reach out and cry out for help. God heard my cry and rescued me. Your trauma may not have been your fault, but pursuing God for healing is your responsibility. You've been hurt, but we can all heal because we have a good God—a great God. And so I want you to have hope. You can be healed, and you can find your strength in community and in Christ.

Why don't we pray together?

Prayer

God, thank you that you are the Father of all compassion, the One who comforts us so that we can comfort others. And we ask for your presence to do what only you can do. Will you give us the courage to start by just acknowledging that we've been hurt and wounded? We may not know how to label our trauma, but we know we need your help.

And so, God, give us a safe community, friends to heal with, trusted Christian counselors to help us process our pain. And we give you our hurt, our confusion, our anger, our guilt, our shame, our doubts, and our rage. We cast our cares on you. And somehow, God, we have the faith to believe that you can make us stronger and able to help others with the same comfort you've given us. We pray this in Jesus' name, amen.

For Reflection

1. Have you acknowledged your trauma to God or to your community? What is your first step to doing that?
2. Have you ever tried counseling or therapy to help deal with your trauma? How has that worked for you? If not well, do you need to find a safer, better place for help? What is your first step for doing that?
3. Do you know anyone who's battling the pain of trauma? If so, will you take a moment to pray for them and perhaps text them with encouragement?

10

Gen Z Will Be Suicide Free

Our Stay Here team has a big vision to stop suicide around the globe, especially for Gen Z. So now I want the good fruit to speak for itself through some stories of how God is setting captives free from self-harm, depression, anxiety, trauma, and suicide. I know all these people personally, and I thank them for being brave enough to tell their story.

These are all accounts of victory, signs that hope is rising all across the country for Americans as well as for people all across the world. And I know that what God did for these friends, He can do for you and anyone who desperately needs life.

God Rewrote My Story
Ciara Cloud

I once found comfort in the idea of disappearing, with the idea of staining myself until I blended in with what broke me.

But someone once told me our testimonies are like works of art, and now I believe mine would be stained glass in a chapel window, the etching of color on a once-clear mirror.

I wanted to disappear when I was sexually assaulted at three, when my home life got rough, when my cousin died from cancer after people prayed for a miraculous healing, and when I thought partying was my only way to be seen. But sometimes when you think you want to disappear, all you really want is to be found.

I grew up in church with a family that loved God but struggled to show me what love is. As a child, I was diagnosed with an anxiety disorder, and because I was too shy to make a name for myself, I became the names everyone else gave me. But I wanted nothing more than to be seen. So when I switched schools, all summer I watched videos on how to become extroverted and attract people. I was desperate for affirmation that I was enough, writing down my goal to become popular so people who had never even met me would message me with "Happy Birthday!" I saw this kind of popularity as my saving grace and quickly found I needed to conform to what popular people did.

Truthfully, I wanted to rebel. I thought living in sin would show the people who had hurt me that they should feel ashamed about how I ended up as a result of their actions. I passed the blame to them instead of processing my feelings. I knew it wasn't healing, but it's what I thought I wanted. I got affirmation from partying, from living for the world, and I began to believe that the "I'm so proud of you" comments I got were everything I'd been searching for. My self-awareness alarms had turned off.

Months after living this way, I did receive those texts on my birthday. Then I went to a party where a drunk girl looked at me and said, "One day you'll find your people." I left angered, thinking I already had. But the feeling I'd waited for my entire life—the validation I'd imagined—was really just a numbness like everything else.

The next week I went to a coffee shop with some people, and a man I didn't know walked in. He stood on a chair proclaiming the gospel, and I'll never forget how I laughed at him as his "fairy tale" became the topic of our table conversation.

That next fall, I got stuck in a love triangle where both guys—one claiming to be a Christian, the other an atheist—said I needed to choose between them. And each one also said I'd have to do sexual things to be in a relationship with him. Somehow smoking, drinking, partying, cussing—none of that bothered me. But because I was having flashbacks to my past sexual assault, I didn't want either of them to have that power over me. God basically used an awful childhood memory to protect me from greater breakage, even when I wasn't living in His will. This was the first time I truly prayed out of desperation, and it went something like, *God, if you're real, show me what a real man of God looks like.*

Then one day I was scrolling on TikTok and saw a guy preaching the gospel. He had his snapchat in the bio, and I added him. We began talking, and I was amazed at how my prayers were answered. He introduced me to a Zoom Bible study group and Snapchat groups, and suddenly my media was filled with online Christian communities.

Over the next few years, I began to teach and speak online about what the gospel was doing in my life. I hadn't seen many women do this, but I found myself with free time and an abundance of isolation during the COVID-19 pandemic, and God can use any yes. I began to forgive the people in my past and work through my relationships with my family, and I even baptized my oldest brother and cousin. I got to become for others what I'd wanted other people to be for me.

People now message me not to wish me a happy birthday but wanting to know who God is. I do street evangelism just like the man who came into that coffee shop. I speak on the very things I used to let speak over me. I learned that pain, abuse, striving—none of that had to be the end of my story. To clean my own stained glass, I needed God, who restored every color. Romans 2:29 says, "A person with a changed heart seeks praise from God, not from people" (NLT).

Disappearing doesn't remove pain; it just removes the possibility of hope. And my testimony isn't wrapped up. I'm waiting on the Lord to come through on some things I can't yet speak about, but this is how I found Him: I sought Him with all my heart.

I know who writes my story, and through Him, I live on promises no person can break.

Social handles: Insta @heyits.cia; TikTok @heyitscia

The Flowers Dried—and I Lived

Claire

I literally had a timeline to end my life in two weeks. I went to the grocery store and bought some purple and pink flowers. Then into the water I poured the contents of the little packet that's supposed to keep flowers alive longer, telling myself, *These are the only beautiful things left in my life, and when they die, it will be my time to go too.*

That night I made a list of everyone I would write a letter to, packed a bag, and left for a Gen Z for Jesus event. I was just hopeless. I had told God, *I'm done. It's over. I can't keep striving and striving. I've got nothing left to give. Where are you?* But He told me, *Just give me one day.* So I did, and the next day at Gen Z for Jesus absolutely changed my life.

First, I realized I wasn't actually saved, so I accepted Jesus. And that was the first day in as long as I could remember that I didn't feel like I wanted to die. I physically felt that weight lift off me during the worship set. And then one of the event people hugged me. I felt the love of God for the first time ever, and it broke me.

Long story short, after the weekend, I got home, and those dang flowers were perfectly dried. They didn't die; they were preserved as if God was telling me, *Your symbol of death and hopelessness will never come to pass. You have meaning in your life.*

I now have those flowers taped to my bulletin board so they're the first thing I see when I wake up in the morning. I am alive. I am alive in Christ. I even got re-baptized into my complete acceptance of Jesus.

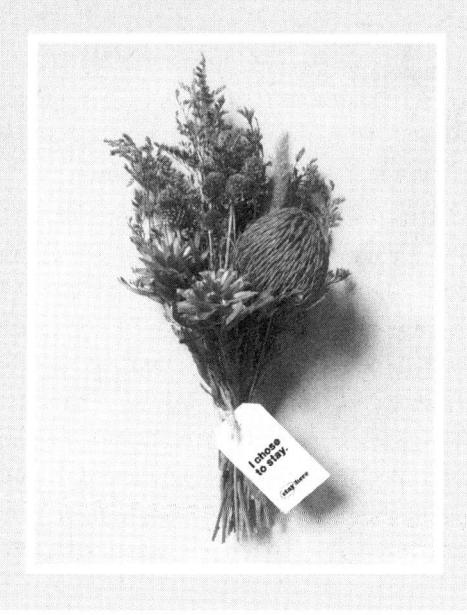

I Found Jesus on TikTok
Camilla Rose

I shared this very testimony with Jacob Coyne at Gen Z for Jesus, a gathering declaring that Gen belongs to Jesus and will be suicide free by the blood of the Lamb.

I grew up with a rocky belief in God. My parents were raised Catholic, but my dad became an atheist, and my mother was "spiritual." My grandparents on my mom's side, however, became Christians and gave us a dose of God every opportunity they had.

I only faintly remember Sunday school, my first story Bible, and the "Now I lay me down to sleep" prayer, but God has shown Himself so faithful even while my trust in Him was so dim.

In 2019, my family decided to move to Texas with no particular reason other than for a bigger house and better weather. During this season of moving and building our home, I experienced heavy oppression with thoughts of death. Then in March 2020, COVID-19 hit, and I came to my end. I was so empty and felt so purposeless, yet I was so spiritually hungry. I struggled with self-harm for months, ripping apart what God had beautifully made and desired to dwell in.

In April 2020, the week I was going to take my life, I encountered something that would forever change me. I opened TikTok as I usually did in the morning, and the first video that showed up was Jacob Coyne asking to pray for me to encounter Jesus. The caption of this video was "Let me show you that God is real," and this is what my soul truly longed for—to know this Living God people proclaimed was the healer and loved me.

That very day He did just that—healed me. God showed Himself to me in an encounter I cannot deny. After I prayed lying on my bed, the love of God flushed over every fear and desire for death, and cultivated such hope in my soul that can come only from Him.

Then on June 6, at twelve years old, I gave my life to Jesus in secret, yet I tried to share about this divine experience through little things like playing worship music and asking my parents for a Bible. In July, I was set on fire to preach the gospel on TikTok, and I would stay up till 3:00 a.m. reading the Bible and talking about whatever the Lord put on my heart. In August, the church right next to our neighborhood opened up again, and we started going there.

On September 6, I was led to get baptized. For months I prayed for my family to come to truly know Jesus, and on October 4 we reached the promised land. We went to a worship event, and that very night, the Holy Spirit fell so powerfully upon my family that we all began to weep and surrender. My mom and sister were baptized that night, and a new fire was overtaking my soul. I was commissioned. By the Holy Spirit I began to be bold in my faith, preaching, holding Bible studies in our home, and living life in prayer and the Scriptures.

A big awakening took place in the months to come. I held a Bible study for my thirteenth birthday, and my neighbors started to be drawn to the Lord by His Spirit. They began to go to church and seek God after years of ignoring Him.

God can do anything with your weak and simple yes to Him. You were made for such a time as this.

The Darkness of Depression
Elijah Lamb

I saw no light to look forward to, no light that could expel the shadows from my heart. My thoughts and feelings were dark. They were vivid, they were heavy, and they were brutal.

Truth be told, I felt attacked on every side and utterly defenseless. Even as a follower of Jesus, I constantly had these suicidal ideations, experiencing the awful back-and-forth between panic and apathy, thinking the total lifelessness I wandered this world with was just a part of the weight I had to bear. I struggled to imagine that Jesus would ever really want to help me or comfort me or heal me, because I believed I had failed Him. I remember weeping through Psalm 13, begging God to come back from wherever He had left me to go.

One particularly difficult night, that poem of David was so heartbreaking to me. I had been sitting alone, weeping in my room, and now it was two or three in the morning. The internal battle was louder than usual, and I was stuck between two options: trying to sleep it off or taking my own life.

I chose the latter and recounted that psalm as I sped down the interstate. At some point I started screaming at God—not *to* Him, *at* Him. I gave Him what I guess could be considered my closing remarks. I was going to fly right off that interstate and finally be done with the fighting.

And then my mind went totally silent. My expression went blank. My tears were dried. My heartbeat slowed. To this day I can't tell you exactly what happened, but it was as though God had simply said "No." I went home and slept like nothing had ever happened.

That wasn't the end of my journey—not by a long shot. But it's one of many moments I look back on with thankfulness. I'm so grateful that God did *whatever* He did. I'm alive because He said no to my goodbye. He saw all the good I've found since then ahead of time and made sure I'd see it too. When I was on the verge of giving up, God wouldn't let me, because He was nowhere near done with me.

At the time I was so blinded by that internal darkness, but now I can look back with clarity and see how Jesus never stopped holding on to me. No matter what I did, the goodness of God stayed hot on my tail. He was always right there. And He's always right there for you too.

I write this to you now through tears. Not ones of sorrow or despair, though I still see those every now and again, but ones of matchless gratitude. I cannot tell you how thankful I am that Jesus made me stay, and I'm certain He's been overjoyed to help me find victory by His blood. Jesus has restored all things for me. He has been my gentle, tender, kind, sweet, wonderful Counselor.

Thanks to Jesus, I am full of joy. My joy is the fruit of His Spirit. My joy is the product of salvation. My joy is His joy made complete in me. Thanks to Jesus, I am full of peace, and my peace surpasses all understanding. My peace comes from my Prince. My peace is His peace. Thanks to Jesus, I am full of hope. My hope is in the hands that make all things good. My hope looks forward to my returning King. My hope is His hope.

There is no place Jesus can be where He won't change everything, and your heart is at the top of His list. The light is coming!

Now I'm Free

Nicolle Belieny

On July 12, 2022, I had already prepared a note and had a plan. Over text, I would tell everyone I knew *Hey, I love you* and see if anyone responded in the next minute. If no one did, then if the first video I found on TikTok told me not to end it all, I would stay. If it didn't, I was ready. I had already strapped a belt onto a pull-up bar I own, and I planned to end it all in the next two minutes.

I texted everyone, but no one responded in that minute I'd allowed. So I opened TikTok, and one of Jacob Coyne's videos was the first one on my For You page. He was talking about how much God loves me, about how God has a plan for me, and I immediately knew this was my sign to stay.

I was struggling with feeling loved because my boyfriend, who had been my best friend of eight years, had just cheated on me. Also, so many negative words were being spoken over me by people from school and even by family members. But because I received affirmation that God loves me and I heard a message specifically about not ending my life, I knew I was seen by God and had a purpose.

Freedom from Loneliness and Suicide

Yasmin Bragatto

For a big chunk of my life, I struggled with a severe feeling of loneliness. It was a kind of loneliness I couldn't ignore by watching a movie. One I couldn't satisfy by simply surrounding myself with people. It was a lingering feeling that seemed ingrained within me.

Everywhere I went, this chronic lonesome feeling plagued me. I grew up in a pretty violent and dysfunctional home, and as a child I began to lose myself in the chaos. I often felt overlooked and misunderstood. By the time I was eleven years old, I was so used to feeling invisible that I think at some point I started to intentionally try to be as unnoticeable as possible.

At school, my teachers and peers might have described me as the class clown or as outgoing and way too talkative.

But as soon as I got home, I found any way I could to make myself disappear. All I wanted was to stop existing. I told myself maybe dying would feel less lonely than being alive.

By age thirteen, I'd established a genuine longing to die. I'd fallen into a deep state of depression, and no one knew—or they did but didn't care enough to help. Many times I'd sit on the bathroom floor late at night sobbing while trying to talk myself out of ending it all. Everything felt dull, and the longer I lived, the less pleasure I found in being alive. I lost every passion, gave up every ambition, and was numb toward any feeling of love. I was so desperate to feel anything at all that I even fell into a habit of self-harm.

As time went on, I developed behavioral patterns that were a clear cry for attention. I used my body for male validation and always tried to make my personality the biggest in the room. All because deep down I was a lonely girl trying to suppress the constant urge to kill herself.

This went on for years. Every day the main thing on my mind was death. I had created several plans, marking several dates, but each time, something in me insisted on my sticking around. Yet nothing within those five years of suicidal torment could pull me out. No antidepressant, no boy, no high, no alcohol. No matter what I tried, I always woke up wishing I hadn't.

Until, alone in my room, I was met with an overwhelming, indescribable love, and His name is Jesus. I still remember my first time reading about what He did on the cross and finally seeing His true character. He wasn't the guy I'd read about on picket signs and Twitter threads. I sobbed uncontrollably because I was overcome with a love I'd never known. When I came to God, I was filled with bitterness and doubt, but He didn't seem to be intimidated by any of that. I said out loud, "If this is who you are, I never want to live for anything else."

> From that moment on, a light of hope I can't ignore has been stored deep within me. Even during my hardest times, suicide stopped being an option because I was made aware of the purpose behind my every breath. Jesus does this cool thing where He restores all that was once stolen from you and redeems all that was once lost. When I was younger, I longed to be seen, loved, and protected, and now Jesus has provided all of that to me in abundance and in ways I never would have received from anyone else.
>
> I tell people finding Jesus was like being able to breathe for the first time or seeing color in a world that was once gray. I was always walking around as a shell of a person, defined by what was done to me, weighed down by my sickness, until I was comforted by the Father, who had always chased after me. Even when I didn't know Him and wanted nothing to do with Him, He still chose me. And He relentlessly chased after my heart until He had me. I have always been irreplaceable to Him.
>
> And when I rest in the arms of a Dad like that, I taste real freedom and know real peace. I have lived suicide free for three years now, and that's only because of the burning love our God has for me.

Final Thoughts

As you can see, all these amazing people within Gen Z were healed in different ways. They all come from different backgrounds, and they all carried different kinds of pain on their backs. God was clearly with them in their pain, and He led them out of it and into freedom in unique ways.

The sad reality, though, is that some messaging has kept a lot of Gen Z bound in the shadows and suffering in silence. I grew up with teaching that said if I just speak to a thing and have enough faith, the thing must move. I was taught that to take authority over unclean spirits means they must bow. That's good, but not every negative emotion is due to evil spirits.

In principle, that all seemed to align with what it means to have the keys to the kingdom, but in practice, it left everything up to me and in my hands. I would bind the spirit of depression over and over again. I would cast out anxiety and renounce my allegiance with fear. Yet I was still plagued with all those things. I was following the template and methods perfectly, but was I still doing something wrong?

As I've matured in the Lord, I've not only come to realize this truth but found safety in it: *Our healing and process for healing is ultimately up to God, not us.* God wants to heal us, but the way He heals might look different from what we expected. He can't be put in a box, and He doesn't heal only one way.

Sometimes Jesus healed people with one touch, and other times He required those who needed healing to push through crowds and reach out to touch Him. Jesus immediately and supernaturally delivered me from many sin patterns and issues over the years; one day I was bound, and the next day I was free. But to receive healing from my depression and anxiety, he required me to reach out my hand.

Reaching out your hand can be allowing Jesus to guide you into a therapist's office or into a doctor's office for medication. Or it can be allowing Him to guide you into community. When we reach out our hand for healing, our faith is in God, not in the method. He will be with you through whatever method He leads you to.

Allow God to lead you in the way you should go, and be free from any shame you've been carrying along the way. He really does want to heal you, and He really can set you free. Will you choose to trust him? To follow Him along His path toward what He has for you? Let Him make you whole. If you do, I believe you will soon have a story to tell much like the ones you just read. God is with you right now, and He's more than willing to heal you from the inside out.

Know this: I'm praying for you, and my email and Instagram are always open if you want to talk. In the meantime, if you're having thoughts of suicide, I hope the pages in this book have given you newfound purpose and a reason to stay here. Reach out and let me know if they have, because that's the only reason I wrote this book. I wrote it thinking about what I would have needed to hear in 2018 when I was in a dark place of pain and trauma, and if you've been in a pit lately, I pray the Lord pulls you out and brings you into your purpose as well.

Prayer

God, I'm letting you out of the box I've put you in. Heal me and make me whole in any way you choose. Jesus, I will follow you into the pathway of freedom. Please remove the shame I've been carrying, the shame false religion has put on me. I know you can heal me, and I'm ready for the process, whether it's instant or over the next few seasons of my life.

Lord, I also pray that Gen Z and every generation following will be suicide free, in the name of Jesus. Use me to save lives. Make me your hands and feet. Send me to the brokenhearted. I want to carry your message into the messiest places and watch your light drown out the darkness. Thank you for the hope you have for me and my generation. The best is yet to come! Amen.

For Reflection

1. What story do you have to tell that can inspire hope in a hurting soul? With whom can you share your story?
2. How have you put God in a box when it comes to the method He may use to heal you, and how has that kept you from reaching out for healing?
3. Will you do what you can for the well-being of those around you? If so, please take Stay Here's free suicide prevention training online and be certified to save lives: www.stayhere.live/acttraining.

Personal Prayer Starters

Insomnia

Dear God, I invite your presence into this place. Fill the atmosphere with your mighty angels. There is no one like you, and I know you're here with me. As the enemy tries to rob me of sleep, please rescue me from his attacks. You never sleep nor slumber, and that means you will watch over me as I sleep. I put my trust in you to end any sleeplessness. In Jesus' name, amen.

If you lie down, you will not be afraid; when you lie down, your sleep will be sweet.

Proverbs 3:24

In peace I will both lie down and sleep; for you alone, O Lord, make me dwell in safety.

Psalm 4:8

Anxiety

Lord, I thank you for drawing near to me when I draw near to you. To think that you are mindful of me overwhelms my soul. But today my spirit is heavy and my body is weak. I can't bear the weight of this anxiety any longer. I recognize I can't get through this alone, and I pray against the very active enemy who is trying to shake my faith and keep my eyes off you. Help me stand strong in you. Strengthen these weary bones and remind me of the truth that this pain and panic will not last forever. It will pass.

Fill me with your joy, peace, and perseverance, Father. Restore my soul and break the chains of anxiety that bind me. I trust you with my panic, and I know that you have the power to take it all away. But even if you don't, I know I don't have to be a slave to my fear. I can rest in the shadow of your wings, and I will rise and overcome by your unwavering strength. In Jesus' name, amen.

Do not be anxious about anything, but in everything by prayer and supplication with thanksgiving let your requests be made known to God. And the peace of God, which surpasses all understanding, will guard your hearts and your minds in Christ Jesus.

Philippians 4:6–7

Depression

I feel lost. Find me, Lord. Pull me up from the waters I'm drowning in so I can breathe again. I feel abandoned. Embrace me, and cover my wounds with your healing love so I can stand restored. I feel trapped.

Break the chains, Lord. Release me from the weights that drag me down. Release me from this prison cell of pain. Come bring your freedom and hope. I'm desperate, yet I seek you, God—the One who conquered the darkness, the One who rose from the dead, the One who can deliver me from this depression—I feel lost, yet I am found in your light. I feel abandoned, yet you are beside me. I feel trapped, yet you call me out of the pit. I feel desperate, yet you lead me to peace and you have all the answers. I choose to put my faith in you above my own feelings. I draw near to you, Lord Jesus. Amen.

It is the LORD who goes before you. He will be with you; he will not leave you or forsake you. Do not fear or be dismayed.

Deuteronomy 31:8

I have said these things to you, that in me you may have peace. In the world you will have tribulation. But take heart; I have overcome the world.

John 16:33

The LORD is near to the brokenhearted and saves the crushed in spirit.

Psalm 34:18

Anger

God, your peace surpasses all my understanding. When anger rises within me, please calm my mind and soothe my heart with your gentle words of life. Fill my whole life with your perfect peace. May my entire personality be shaped by your peace rather than by my frustration.

With your Holy Spirit in my life, I can overcome anger. Help me reflect your character, being slow to anger and quick to love. Look upon me and cause your face to shine upon me. Help me let go and forgive. Through Jesus Christ I pray, amen.

Know this, my beloved brothers: let every person be quick to hear, slow to speak, slow to anger; for the anger of man does not produce the righteousness of God. Therefore put away all filthiness and rampant wickedness and receive with meekness the implanted word, which is able to save your souls.

James 1:19–21

But you, O Lord, are a God merciful and gracious, slow to anger and abounding in steadfast love and faithfulness.

Psalm 86:15

Salvation

Dear God, I come before you today with a humble heart, and I surrender my life to you. I believe that Jesus Christ was born free of sin, lived a sinless and perfect life, died on a cross to save me from my own sin, and rose three days later. I believe in your gift of salvation and eternal life because of the sacrifice of Jesus Christ.

God, today I repent and turn from my old way of life. Because of your mercy and grace, I can have childlike faith. Today I ask for new life through Jesus Christ and the power of the Holy Spirit. Thank you, God, for forgiving me and making me brand-new. In Jesus' name, amen.

If you confess with your mouth that Jesus is Lord and believe in your heart that God raised him from the dead, you will be saved. For with the heart one believes and is justified, and with the mouth one confesses and is saved. . . . For "everyone who calls on the name of the Lord will be saved."

Romans 10:9–10, 13

For by grace you have been saved through faith. And this is not your own doing; it is the gift of God, not a result of works, so that no one may boast. For we are his workmanship, created in Christ Jesus for good works, which God prepared beforehand, that we should walk in them.

Ephesians 2:8–10

Stay Here Resources

- Hopeline Live Chat 24/7: www.thehopeline.com/gethelp/
- Stay Here clothing: www.stayhere.store
- Get certified to prevent suicide. Take our free online training: www.stayhere.live/acttraining
- Join the Stay Here team: www.stayhere.live/joinourteam
- Join the movement to help save lives today. Text "stay here" to (253) 243-2771.
- Donate to the cause: www.stayhere.live/donate
- Book Jacob Coyne to speak at your church, school, or event: www.stayhere.live/bookjacobcoyne

Acknowledgments

Jonah Coyne, you're the best brother and friend I could ever ask for. I love you. I'm so glad that after all these years, we're still running after the Lord just as we did at the start. I'll always believe in you and stand with you, heart and soul.

David Campbell, you helped me process my pain and led me to the light when all I felt was darkness and fear. Thank you for all your wisdom.

Gabriel Wilson, you're my covenant brother and friend. I'm so grateful for the laughter we've shared together and the tears we've shed in your recording studio. Thanks for sitting with me and listening.

Terra Shmidtke, you're the best mom. I'm so grateful for the way God has moved in our relationship and made it what it is today. I love you, and I miss you every single day. Thanks for being the first one to believe in Stay Here and sow into it and my family.

Acknowledgments

Chad Coyne, thank you for leading me to Jesus. I wouldn't be here if you hadn't made the leap first. I love you, Dad.

Special thanks to the team at Chosen Books for believing in this project and making a dream become a reality. David Sluka, thanks for reaching out and making this happen.

Notes

Chapter 1 This Is Your Sign to Live

1. Suicide Statistics, "2021 USA General Statistics," SAVE, https://save.org/about-suicide/suicide-statistics/.

2. "How to Speed Read a Business Book in 90 Minutes," SCORO, https://www.scoro.com/blog/how-to-speed-read-a-business-book/.

3. Marco Margaritoff, edited by John Kuroski, "Inside the Text of Kurt Cobain's Heartwrenching Suicide Note," ati, January 2, 2020, https://allthatsinteresting.com/kurt-cobain-suicide-note.

4. Jennifer Michael Hecht, "How the media covers celebrity suicides can have life-or-death consequences," Vox, updated June 8, 2018, https://www.vox.com/first-person/2018/5/5/17319632/anthony-bourdain-kate-spade-cause-of-death-suicide-celebrities-reporting.

Chapter 3 It's Okay to Not Be Okay, but It's Not Okay to Stay That Way

1. Porn Industry Archives, Enough Is Enough, https://enough.org/stats_porn_industry_archives.

2. Daniel Ruby, "36 TikTok Statistics 2023: How Many Users Are There!," January 20, 2023, DEMAND SAGE, https://www.demandsage.com/tiktok-user-statistics/.

3. Ryan Faughnder, "Gen Z spends half its waking hours on screen time," *Los Angeles Times*, April 12, 2022, https://www.latimes.com/entertainment-arts/business/newsletter/2022-04-12/gen-z-spends-half-its-waking-hours-on-screen-time-heres-the-good-and-bad-news-for-hollywood-the-wide-shot.

4. "Mental Illness," National Institute of Mental Health, https://www.nimh.nih.gov/health/statistics/mental-illness.

5. Shannon Firth, "Teen Suicides Jump 29% Over the Past Decade, Report Finds," MedPage Today, October 12, 2022, https://www.medpagetoday.com/psychiatry/generalpsychiatry/101188.

6. "KSHB, Suicide Rates High in Middle-Aged White Men," St. Luke's, September 21, 2022, https://www.saintlukeskc.org/about/news/kshb-suicide-rates-high-middle-aged-white-men.

7. Suicide Statistics, American Foundation for Suicide Prevention, https://afsp.org/suicide-statistics/.

Chapter 5 When Anxiety Attacks

1. Charles Spurgeon, sermon, "The Saddest Cry from the Cross," https://www.thekingdomcollective.com/spurgeon/sermon/2803/.

2. Charles Spurgeon, sermon, "Night—and Jesus Not There!" https://www.thekingdomcollective.com/spurgeon/sermon/2945/.

3. Michael Reeves, *Spurgeon on the Christian Life: Alive in Christ*, citing Charles Ray, "The Life of Susannah Spurgeon" in *Morning Devotions by Susannah Spurgeon: Free Grace and Dying Love* (Edinburgh: Banner of Truth, 2006), 166.

4. James Hamblin, "Anorexia and the 'Too Fat to Walk Through the Door' Experiment," *The Atlantic*, June 12, 2013, https://www.theatlantic.com/health/archive/2013/06/anorexia-and-the-too-fat-to-fit-through-the-door-experiment/276790/.

5. "Catastrophizing," *Psychology Today*, https://www.psychologytoday.com/us/basics/catastrophizing.

6. Don Joseph Goewey, contributor, "80 Percent of What We Worry About Never Happens," HUFFPOST, December 6, 2017, https://www.huffpost.com/entry/85-of-what-we-worry-about_b_8028368.

Chapter 7 The Prison Cell of Anger

1. Lewis B. Smedes, *Forgive and Forget: Healing the Hurts We Don't Deserve* (San Francisco: HarperCollins, 1984).

2. Ellen Diamond, "The Links Between Your Mental and Physical Health," Psychreg, updated April 9, 2022, https://www.psychreg.org/links-between-mental-health-physical-health/.

Chapter 8 Stuck in the Loop of Stinking Thinking

1. Jason Murdock, "Humans Have More than 6,000 Thoughts per Day, Psychologists Discover," *Newsweek*, July 15, 2020, https://www.newsweek.com/humans-6000-thoughts-every-day-1517963.

2. "Positive thinking: Stop negative self-talk to reduce stress," Mayo Clinic, https://www.mayoclinic.org/healthy-lifestyle/stress-management/in-depth/positive-thinking/art-20043950.

Chapter 9 Jesus Can Heal Your Trauma

1. "Trauma," Merriam-Webster's Dictionary, https://www.merriam-webster.com/dictionary/trauma.

Jacob Coyne was born and raised in Tacoma, Washington. Even though he grew up in a Christian home, his teenage years were full of rebellion as he gave in to teen angst and peer pressure. One day in 2009, Jacob had a life-changing encounter with Jesus Christ. His father, Chad, brought him and his brother, Jonah, to a men's Bible study and prayer group, where Jacob was instantly and radically delivered from his licentious and sinful lifestyle and filled with the Holy Spirit.

After encountering the love and power of the real Jesus, Jacob decided to dedicate the rest of his life to following Him and telling the world all about Him through preaching, teaching, and praying for the sick.

In 2013, Jacob met his wife, Mariah, at the church where they both worked as youth and worship pastors. They've been happily married since 2014. After working together at the same church in their hometown for six years, the Coynes made one of the biggest decisions of their lives by resigning and moving forward into what the Lord was calling them to next. In 2020, they founded Stay Here, a nonprofit mental health organization that trains and equips people to stop suicide and help heal the brokenhearted.

Jacob is a revivalist, preacher, visionary, and social media creative as well as a husband and father. Along with raising his three daughters—River Jordan, Lively Grace, and Holly Evangeline—with his wife in Tennessee, he is the director of Stay Here and spends a quarter of the year traveling to churches and schools to preach the gospel of Jesus and spread His message of hope.

Jacob believes that Jesus is the same yesterday, today, and forever and that everyone can encounter Him in the exact same way we see sinners, tax collectors, and the sick encountering Him in the Gospels of Matthew, Mark, Luke, and John. Jacob passionately lives out his purpose to win souls for Christ and to stop suicide across the globe.

Follow Jacob:
@jacobcoyne
@jacobcoyne

Contact him:
Online (for booking): www.stayhere.live
Email: jacob@stayhere.live